OVERCOME NECK & BACK PAIN

KIT LAUGHLIN

A Fireside Book
Published by Simon & Schuster

FIRESIDE
Rockefeller Center
1230 Avenue of the Americas
New York, NY 10020

First published in 1995 by BodyPress

First Fireside Edition 1998
Published by arrangement with Simon & Schuster Australia

FIRESIDE and colophon are registered trademarks
of Simon & Schuster

Designed by Jeremy Mears. Http://announce.com/~jeremy

Manufactured in the United States of America

10 9 8 7 6 5 4 3 2 1

Library of Congress Cataloging-in-Publication Data is available.

ISBN 0-684-85252-7

To my mother and my father

For Olivia

MEDICAL DISCLAIMER

This publication contains the opinions and ideas of its author. It is intended to provide helpful and informative material on the subjects addressed in the publication. It is sold with the understanding that the author and publisher are not engaged in rendering medical, health, psychological or any other kind of personal professional services in the book. If the reader requires personal medical, health or other assistance or advice, a competent professional should be consulted.

The author and publisher specifically disclaim all responsibility for any liability, loss or risk, personal or otherwise, which is incurred as a consequence, directly or indirectly, of the use and application of any of the contents of this book.

CONTENTS

ILLUSTRATIONS

WHY THE INTEREST IN NECK AND BACK PAIN?

It seems that everyone has suffered neck or back pain at some stage. Neck or back pain affects between 60% and 85% of people. Probably you are one of these people. In one study, researchers reported that 21% of patients experienced back pain in the 14 days preceding the study. Another study reported that at least 5% of all patient visits to the doctor are due to back pain.

Tremendous costs are involved. Neck and back pain account for half the worker's compensation payments in the United States and Australia, they are the single greatest cause of lost work time in both countries, and low back pain alone costs over $85 billion annually in the United States, about one-third of this amount being the direct costs of medical care. The 10% or so of patients who suffer chronic back pain account for 75% of Australia's rehabilitation and compensation payments. The social cost cannot be calculated—back pain is the most frequent cause of inactivity among people under 45 years of age. In the U.S., Great Britain and Australia, the number of people disabled by these problems has increased exponentially since the 1970s, during a period of only modest population increase (Schwarzer, 1996; Rainville *et al.*, 1996).

However, patients are not the only ones to suffer. Back pain has been described as "a wilderness across whose inhospitable terrain orthopedic surgeons, neurosurgeons, physiotherapists and, above all, general practitioners are doomed to travel" (Littler, 1983). Most doctors believe "there is little doubt that most cases are due to derangement of the intervertebral joint in association with 'degeneration' of the disc and arthrosis of the facet joints" (Ganora, 1984), or, as it was put more simply, "more than 95% of patients with low back pain suffer from mechanical back pain" (Schwarzer, 1996, p. 108). And yet an article in the *New York Times* about a study published in the *New England Journal of Medicine* raises serious doubts about these claims: nearly two-thirds of a group studied had "spinal abnormalities, including bulging or protruding discs, herniated discs, and degenerated discs"—but none of the subjects in the study had back pain, or ever had suffered from this problem (Kolata, 1994).

What is this book about?

I have found that most neck and back pain is experienced in the muscles associated with the spine. The pain is caused by excessive tension held in these muscles and is the result of a variety of causes, from structural imbalances to various aspects of lifestyle. These causes can be treated. Except for a very small percentage of neck and back pain which can be dealt with successfully by surgery or drug therapy, I advocate a conservative, exercise-based approach, the subject of this book.

What can I do?

My approach to overcoming neck and back pain has two parts. The first step is to help you identify which muscles are involved in your particular problem and to teach you the most efficient ways to relieve this excess tension, using extremely efficient stretching exercises, initially to be done only twice per week. This phase of treatment (the *rehabilitation* phase) is enhanced by teaching you how to use *directed relaxation* to assist the body to sleep and to enhance its healing tendencies.

The second step (the *prevention* phase) conditions all of the relevant parts of the body by using more advanced stretching exercises and later, by adding specific strengthening exercises, to provide a measure of protection for the future. In these two chapters, I shall present an approach to neck and back pain that is effective in practical terms and a later chapter considers the problem in theoretical terms, and will help you to make sense of the conflicting research on the problem.

Who should use this book?

This book is written for anyone who suffers recurring neck or back pain, or who wishes to avoid these problems. Recovery isn't quick or simple, but there aren't many other options either. Unless your back or neck problem is of the kind that can be treated effectively by surgery or drug therapy (probably less than 10% of the cases presented to general practitioners), you may have found that the range of options seems limited to avoidance of the activity thought to be the cause or treatment of the symptoms. If treatment is successful, your back will be returned to normal; that is, to its "preinjury" level of function—consequently, there is no guarantee that the problem will not return. My aim is to present a unified and comprehensive self-help approach. For those fortunate enough not to have such problems, the approach will increase the suppleness and strength of your neck and back to reduce the likelihood of injury to these areas.

How this book is set out

The introduction sounds a more personal note than following chapters. It begins with a brief history of events which led me to my current approach, including a rather lengthy stay in Japan where I studied *Shiatsu* and a number of traditional exercise systems. I consider the various exercise systems from which I derived my own, the courses called *Posture & Flexibility*, and *Strength & Flexibility*, currently taught at the Australian National University. My clinic in Canberra (the *Shoshin Center*) is mentioned, and I present some relevant neck and back pain case studies. The first three chapters include the self-diagnosis method, and the stretching and strengthening exercises—these are the nuts and bolts of my approach.

Chapter one takes you through the self-diagnosis step-by-step. There is a flow-chart of the diagnosis method at the end of the chapter, and a page to photocopy. On this you fill out the results of the leg length tests and the functional flexibility tests. Fill it in as you go through the chapter. There is also an illustration of where pain may be experienced in the neck and back, and exercises likely to be useful are listed alongside.

Chapter two contains the basic pain-relieving and rehabilitation exercises; the first section describes exercises for the back, and the second describes exercises for the neck. These are the most important exercises in the book, and for most people are the only ones they need to do on a regular basis.

Chapter three details the preventive stretching exercises. These are designed to improve and balance your existing flexibility, and allow you to focus more closely on your problem areas with stronger techniques. The second part of chapter three outlines my approach to strengthening exercise, and details a set of graded strength exercises, from a minimal set suitable for doing at home through to more elaborate exercises for which some equipment is needed.

However, do not go straight to the exercises without reading the cautions section below. Inappropriate exercise may worsen your condition, and the nature of the problem is the best guide to selecting the exercises which are right for you.

You will get more out of the exercises if you have a reasonable working knowledge of the anatomy of the areas of interest. For this reason, useful functional anatomical information will be found together with the exercises. Organizing the book this way means that you do not need to go backwards and forwards between the exercises and the anatomical details upon which the exercises so crucially depend. As mentioned, much experience has shown that the actual locus of neck or back pain tends to be the muscles associated with the spine. As each muscle has a clearly definable function, this knowledge will help you locate the particular group concerned, and guide you to the best exercise. The book has been bound so it can be left open on the floor beside you, to enable you to check your form as you practice, and the practical sections include **Notes** (presented in a larger typeface than the text) that contain the most important details about how to do each exercise. These are arranged alongside the photographs for easy reference.

Chapter four discusses the various causes of neck and back pain, from a number of medical perspectives beginning with that of western medicine. One of the reasons for so doing is that western medicine has the most detailed understanding of anatomy, and this knowledge is fundamental to my approach. Another reason is that we are familiar with the western medical perspective—it is the medicine of our culture. This chapter includes a brief consideration of chiropractic and osteopathy because neck and back pain is the main concern of these practitioners. Oriental medicine and some of the bodywork schools are also considered. Acute and chronic pain are treated separately, and mention is made of additional contributing factors. The chapter sounds a note on the limitations of the very idea of cause with respect to common illnesses, and offers a rationale for my functional approach. The experiences of the workshops we have been running for individuals and practitioners are presented, and consideration is given to choice of beds and pillows.

Chapter five provides a justification for including relaxation techniques as part of the larger approach to overcoming neck and back pain. It discusses practical stress management briefly, outlines the current understanding of stress and its effects on the body, and ends with an easy-to-learn method for relaxation. Useful guided visualization techniques for speeding up the healing process are included in the relaxation script.

Cautions

Before you begin, some notes of caution must be sounded. If you are undergoing some form of treatment at the moment, you must discuss the exercises presented in the book with your practitioner before beginning. It is a matter both of courtesy and safety—some of the exercises may be inappropriate for your condition. Further, embarking on a course of exercises that have not been examined or approved by your practitioner may void any compensation to which you may be entitled. I have written this book in good faith, but I cannot personally supervise your performance of the movements, and therefore cannot accept any responsibility for errors you make. Neither can I know the particular details of a condition you may have—this is your responsibility. These aspects necessitate the greatest caution on your part—the fact that thousands of people have benefited from this system is no guarantee that you will. Consequently you must approach the exercises with caution, and you must monitor the effects closely.

Next, **do not refer only to the photographs.** You must read the sometimes lengthy descriptions that accompany them. Information vital to safety is contained in the text, along with descriptions of how to press or pull certain parts in certain ways. **It is not possible to understand the exercises only by looking at the photographs.**

The next caution concerns the order in which the exercises are presented. In most cases the easiest and safest versions of any movement are shown first; these versions are marked **easiest** in the text. More difficult versions are labeled **intermediate**; the most difficult are labeled **advanced**. This is the order in which you should attempt them. Even if you know that you can do a more difficult version, begin with the easiest one. You can always learn something about the way your body works from doing an easier rather than a more difficult version of an exercise, simply because you can concentrate more on your responses to a movement rather than its complexities. Additionally, the easier versions are a useful warm-up for the later ones.

Lastly, I wish to discuss some practical cautions. Exercise in the evenings rather than the mornings as the body is more supple then. You must not exercise within an hour and a half of eating. It is best to exercise in the hour before you eat the evening meal. Always go to the toilet before beginning. Wear clothing that both keeps you warm, and permits free movement. Some of the exercises require a strap, strong towel, or some other method of holding a part of the body, so have something handy. For the first few weeks or months, I suggest that you stretch only twice a week, which may be increased to three times as you improve. The text includes specific instructions on the few exercises I recommend be done daily to relieve the body of the effects of the day's stress. More of this later.

The following caution may be self-evident, but permit me to labor a vital point. You must imitate the *form* of the exercises demonstrated, not my *performance* of them. The purpose of the precise descriptions and photographs is so that you can place yourself in the positions I have found to produce the best results. You then proceed with the stages of the movements only until you feel the stretch I describe, and **stop at that point.** In the demonstration of the movement, I may have taken the particular limb further in the range of movement than you can, but this is immaterial. (You may well be able to stretch further than I in some exercises, too.) **The sole purpose of an exercise is to feel a stretch in the right place.** Please keep this in mind—most teaching of stretching exercise fails on this crucial point.

The most general, and important, caution I have saved until last. It is that **you must listen to what your body tells you while you are doing the movements**—no one else can do this for you, not even the best teacher. Very early in your practice you must learn the essential difference between the right kind of stretch sensation and going too far. For this reason, I urge you to do too little rather than too much in the beginning—realizing the difference too late will be painful, and possibly dangerous. Remember the old adage: "Rome was not built in a day."

The *Introduction* provides you with the background to the approach advocated in the book. If you prefer, you may go straight to chapter one, the self-diagnosis method, and return to the *Introduction* at a later time.

BACKGROUND TO THE APPROACH

In this introduction, I should like to give you some personal details, which I hope will both be interesting and give you some insight into what led me to develop the methods presented in the rest of the book.

During the early 1980s, I was a television director and a struggling athlete. I trained for the 800- and 1500-meter races, the so-called middle distance events. Directing the Australian Broadcasting Commission's nightly current affairs program *Nationwide* was stressful enough on its own; together with all the running training—we ran 100 miles (160 km) a week in the winter months—I now think that I was asking too much of myself. I used to hold a tremendous amount of tension in the middle back muscles. Despite physiotherapy and chiropractic treatments, the problem never really improved beyond temporary relief.

Some sort of insight occurred one day when I bent down to touch my toes after an interval training session at Sydney University. At full stretch my fingers came a few inches below my knees, and that was with my back bent like a bow. Someone took a photograph of me doing this, and it ended up on the wall at the H. K. Ward gym (where many of the local track and field athletes did their weight training), suitably inscribed "Rubber Man."

The next insight occurred when I was using the seated heel raise machine (from the seated position a padded bar over the knees is lifted by the feet to strengthen *soleus*, one of the two calf muscles). I placed my feet evenly on the footrest and positioned my heels level with each other. One knee contacted the support bar. The other was a full centimeter or so lower. Naturally, my first thought was that the machine had been bent by one of the serious bodybuilders using too much weight. I looked at it carefully, got a tape measure from the attendant at the front desk, and after careful checking decided that it was straight. Only then did the possibility that I might not be straight occur to me. Careful measurement revealed that my right leg from knee to heel was noticeably shorter than my left. I mention this only to highlight the point that we resist the notion that there might be something less than ideal in our own physical makeup, but consideration of all possibly relevant information is essential if we wish to overcome our problems.

Once I had accepted the difference (in fact my right leg is shorter by about three quarters of an inch or two centimeters, evenly divided between the upper and lower leg), I began to think about the effects this structural asymmetry might have caused. I had trained for both Olympic and power lifting for years before losing quite a deal of weight to become a middle distance runner. I realized that years of weight training adapted my body to two major stresses—the stresses of the training itself, and the asymmetric distribution of those forces as resolved in my particular body, so not only had I become extremely tight in the process but had also developed an individual *pattern* of flexibility. I began "limber" classes at a Sydney dance studio, and these patterns became only too clear. I also quickly realized that the approach adopted in these classes was not efficient for teaching adults how to become flexible. The young students were very supple and had become flexible while they were still children. What looked like stretching classes were really preparation, or an extended warmup for their ballet classes later in the day. My experience there made me think about the differences between adults' and children's bodies, and how one might improve on the standard approaches to the problem of how to teach adults to become flexible.

At this time, I experimented with lifts of various thicknesses in my right shoe. The difference it made to running was immediately apparent. The shooting pains in between the shoulder blades experienced in the finishing stretches of my races all but disappeared, and on using the insert the first time, I immediately felt more balanced walking and running.

During the late 1970s I attended yoga classes at various places around Sydney. I found the classes relatively inflexible in their teaching approach: students lined up in neat rows and little dialogue. The strict atmosphere often discouraged questions at the very time one needed assistance. I was disturbed by the tendency for some teachers to accept the pronouncements of their own teachers uncritically. Guru worship was commonplace, and many teachers had adopted the mannerisms and aphorisms of their own gurus. What I subsequently learned to be the correct form of various poses was being distorted by many students in their attempt to imitate the teacher through simple inflexibility. Questions like, "why do we do it this way?" were left unanswered, or deflected with replies like "tradition," or "that's the way the posture is taught by my teacher," and so on. I met few teachers who had more than a passing acquaintance with anatomy—the one aspect of western medicine normally unquestioned by the alternative healing arts. Of course, these were my particular experiences at the time; much has changed since these early days, and anatomical knowledge is now emphasized in contemporary yoga teaching.

During this period I also resumed martial arts training, and so did the kind of stretching usually employed in these arts during the warmup—vigorous dynamic movements, assisted by a partner or an instructor, and all over in 15 minutes before the real training began. No attention was paid to form in the exercises, and I injured myself a number of times using this approach. On one occasion, I pulled a groin muscle (one of the *adductors*) that took nine or ten months to heal and which was subsequently injured at another training session.

I had my thirtieth birthday in Japan. I had had enough of television, and decided to go to the source for martial arts. I was dismayed to find the same approach to stretching used there too. I found disbelief on the part of teachers who could not accept that someone who had trained for ten years or so was not perfectly flexible. They had no effective suggestions on how to become more flexible. They had all done the usual stretching as children (usual in Japan, anyway), started their martial arts training at an early age and consequently did not need to know how to make an adult flexible. The severe training I went through (I was a live-in student, called an *uchi deshi*) made my back muscles even tighter. After nearly a year and a half of this life, I found myself unable to recover from an illness that alternated between a cold and influenza for six months. A friend had been studying a form of oriental medicine for a year or so (*shiatsu*) and, sick of being kept awake at night when I visited, he suggested that I go to see his teacher.

It was a revelation. Never have I let anyone hurt me so much. I was holding a tremendous amount of tension in the muscles of my body, and all the places he worked on, including my back, were incredibly tender to touch. The *sensei* told me that although my body was strong it was holding excessive tension everywhere, which he felt was the result of the stress of the work I used to do plus the effects of the rigorous current training. He would poke my body and say in English, "Too hard, too hard." I confess I was skeptical of a treatment that consisted merely of maintaining a leaning pressure on various places using the elbows and thumbs mainly, together with a few simple stretches and manipulations of the bones of the body. However, I started to feel better that same day, and by the time of the next treatment (a week later) the cold had gone. It was at the conclusion of the second treatment that I was introduced to a woman who would change my way of thinking about flexibility. Ms. K— was a diminutive Japanese woman around 35 years old. She was the translator for the shiatsu classes presented for foreigners at the center. *Sensei* mentioned that I was interested in becoming more flexible. Ms. K—'s way of getting to the floor for this conversation involved sliding through the side splits into front splits, then lifting herself into *seiza*, the normal Japanese way of sitting on one's feet. It certainly got my attention.

Ms. K— and I were to do considerable work together during the ensuing few years on flexibility and shiatsu, as I became a student. She was the sole surviving *shihan* (senior teacher) of an exercise method called *Jikyo Jutsu*. Roughly translated, this means "self-help method." Like *Tai Chi*, it is based on meridian theory, the practice of which is designed to "harmonize energy flow" around the body and promote internal health, in much the same way as shiatsu. This improvement in internal health is said to be responsible for the increase in flexibility that follows. In other words, the acquisition of flexibility was deemed to be a side effect of health. Quite different to our western approach, I thought. The exercises themselves were an interesting mixture of dynamic stretching movements and pressure point therapy. In time I was awarded a *shodan* (a "first degree" black belt). "*Sho*" is the character for "beginning," and unlike other parts of the world where a black belt is often regarded as a pinnacle of achievement, in Japan it signifies a starting point.

Part of the learning process of shiatsu involves receiving treatment from one's teacher. I received treatment for a year or more on a fortnightly basis, did the *Jikyo Jutsu*, and taught and attended yoga classes in Tokyo. By the time I had been in Japan for three years or so, my back felt considerably better and my flexibility was noticeably improved, particularly when I cast my mind back to the "Rubber Man" era. All was progressing, I felt. An incident one day on my way to teaching a stretching class at the well-known "Clark-Hatch" gym in Tokyo soon dispelled my complacency. While walking across the car park (thinking about something else), I inadvertently stepped off a low curb—no more than three or four inches high—and felt a stabbing pain in my lower back. The sensation was so strong it literally took my breath away. I continued walking to the gym, and although my back did not feel "right," I taught the class. When I returned home that evening, I stripped off and looked at myself in the full-length mirror in the bathroom. Unbelievably, my hips seemed displaced so much to one side that the normal indentation of the waist had completely disappeared on one side, compensated for by double the amount on the other. I had trouble accepting the evidence of my eyes; I could not believe what I was seeing.

The following days suggested that this distortion was going to be with me for some time. I had treatment variously from my shiatsu teacher, a well-known local chiropractor, and in desperation yet another shiatsu teacher. None altered the displacement by any extent that I could see or feel. Worse still were their claims that they had not seen any equivalent problem in all their years of practice. I was so worried by this that I travelled four hours north of Tokyo to a famous chiropractor, but he could not help either. Very slowly, with careful stretching over a period of seven or eight weeks, my shape returned to normal. I now think that the incident resulted from an imbalance of too much flexibility and not enough strength, my body being predisposed to certain types of injury due to my leg-length difference.

I spent considerable time thinking about the physical structures involved. One chiropractor suggested that the distortion resulted from one hip bone (the *ilium*) moving with respect to the *sacrum* (in effect, driven upwards by the unexpected force of stepping off the curb onto my shorter leg while completely relaxed). This joint, particularly in men, is normally stable, the ligaments binding the *sacroiliac* joints on both sides of the pelvis are extremely strong, and the internal surfaces of the joint are irregular and fit each other. It is possible that all the hip abduction work (legs-apart stretching) I had been doing had upset the stability of the *pubic symphysis* (the joint where the pubic bones come together at the front of the pelvis), thereby permitting the much more stable sacroiliac joint to move. However, because the shape of the distortion appeared simply to be an extremely exaggerated version of the normal lateral curve in my lumbar spine induced by my leg-length difference, I thought this unlikely. Another chiropractor thought that my pelvis had "rotated" with respect to the lumbar spine, and that was the cause of the problem. When my teacher suggested that enough shiatsu treatment would even up the length of my legs, I felt that I needed to consider the problem in depth.

The apparently conflicting explanations I had been offered for the problem led me to think about possible relationships between information produced in different frameworks, and about standards of evidence. It seemed to me then (and seems so today) that there are various kinds of facts about the world, and that there are different expectations of reliability in relation to these facts. "Information" or "facts" depend crucially on the assumptions underlying the different frameworks giving rise to them, and these facts come bound together with indices of reliability. In this sense there are no certain facts (we might say, though, that some facts are very reliable and others less so), but comparison of explanatory range, assumptions, reliability indices and suitable constraints permit evaluation of different kinds of facts. In respect to my back problem, for example, it was not that one perspective was wrong and another right. Each perspective provided one window on the problem—a window that revealed a particular view.

These musings led me to think that, in respect to a health problem, we might conveniently divide the body into psychological and physical aspects for particular reasons, as western medicine ordinarily does. For example, the physical body might be considered in terms of a spectrum, from its least-alterable to most-alterable substances, as one way of deciding how to tackle a problem. One advantage of working with the physical aspects of a body (in contrast to the psychological) is that some of the cause and effect relationships are better known, and are often measurable. For instance, we know that the nerves of the body react most quickly to stress, followed shortly after by the muscles, then ligaments and tendons, and the slowest to change are the hardest substances in the body—the bones and teeth. How these substances manifest their reactions to particular stressors is well known. Knowing this about the body's organization, in respect to a problem like neck or back pain, we may affect the brain and the nerves using relaxation techniques, we may affect patterns of muscular tension, the results of stress, by using the stretching exercises, and we can strengthen the body in various ways against expected future stress.

This simplified approach may seem like a structural and engineering analysis, but the oriental medical "umbrella" permits useful association of aspects of the problem whose precise causal relationship is not clear. The oriental perspective allows greater freedom than the western medical approach, because it is a medicine of correlation rather than cause—it is a system of correspondence (Porkert, 1974). I will discuss the problems of causality further in chapter four. The essence of my approach is that, in respect of multicausal problems, analysis and treatment is better directed towards a desired *outcome* rather than trying to solve the problems of causality. This approach can avoid the pitfalls of symptomatic treatment.

Shoshin Center

In 1988 I opened the Shoshin Center, specializing in shiatsu. One of the four main forms of oriental medicine in the modern world, shiatsu applies periods of still, manual pressure on the acupuncture points for treatment following the *yin-yang* and the *five element* (or *transformation*) theories. Shiatsu was developed in Japan around the turn of the century by joining aspects of the Palmer chiropractic method with traditional Chinese massage, called *anma* in its Japanese form. Although I opened my center with the intention of practicing preventive medicine, the majority of patients were seeking a cure for a particular problem affecting them at the time. Although I stressed the medium and long-term effectiveness of lifestyle modification and the application of specific exercises for their problems, most patients preferred to return at three- or six-month intervals for treatment. By the end of the first year, it was clear that most patients wanted help with neck and back pain more than any other problems, and this pattern has continued to this day.

At any initial consultation in my clinic, I state that we should both know after a treatment or two whether my approach is likely to be effective, and I stress that any recommended exercise is an integral part of the treatment. It is essential to the success of any treatment that patients take responsibility for their problems. Most patients are agreeably surprised to be so actively involved in the outcome of the treatment. For many, it is a new experience.

Case studies from the clinic

I should like to mention the experiences of a few patients briefly, for they illustrate my method at work and the types of problems for which it might prove helpful.

The first concerns a young (21) male rower. He came to me complaining of back pain caused, he said, by lifting a rowing "shell" (boat) out of the water. These were the only details he gave me. When I examined him, I found a marked *scoliosis* (lateral curvature of the spine), with the right shoulder carried high on the outside of a left-facing concavity. He was right-handed and, as you might expect, the development of the muscles of the right side of the spine was noticeably greater than the left. He rowed on the left side of the boat so that, in addition to the uneven development caused by the scoliosis, he displayed an extra muscular development caused both by being right-handed, and the fact that the right shoulder was moving through a greater arc than the left (due to the rotation that sweep rowing adds to the extension of the basic rowing movement). Although he complained of low back pain when we first spoke, I asked him whether his middle and upper back also troubled him. As this was so, my first suggestion was for him to train on the other side of the boat once or twice a week and to report back.

Turning then to his low back pain, I performed a structural examination and the usual tests of functional flexibility, concentrating on a comparison of left and right, as will be developed below. There were marked differences in all the relevant tests, but no discernible leg-length difference. I enrolled him in a beginners' stretching class, and after a couple of months he reported that the pain had gone. We then embarked on a strengthening program together, and I was fascinated to see that although a nationally competitive rower, he had very poor strength in the trunk muscles. Considering the excellent development of the upper and lower body, I considered it likely that this lack of strength was a contributing cause of his problems, because his waist would not be capable of transmitting the strength of the legs and hips to the arms without distortion. To address this, I developed the basis of the waist strengthening program offered later in this book. After concentrating on the stretching and strengthening exercises for about eight months, he competed in the annual "Nationals" for rowers, recording the third-highest ergometer score without a trace of back pain. Today, some five years later, there has not been any recurrence of the original problem.

The extraordinary aspect of this case was that after the Nationals, the young man's doctor revealed to me that when the rower "hurt his back" the year before while lifting the boat out of the water, he had in fact suffered a "massive extrusion of the L_5-S_1 intervertebral disc, so much so that he had displayed various neurological deficits" at that time. As you will see, *neurological deficits* are considered hard evidence of nerve impingement and serious pathology. Even in the case of demonstrable pathology—of the sort often requiring surgery—the approach I advocated was successful. I realize that this is a highly unusual case and perhaps is evidence only of the superior recuperative capacity of a top athlete. Nonetheless, providing one has the support of one's doctor, I urge a conservative "wait-and-see" approach initially, followed by cautious stretching exercise, and followed up with strengthening exercises as the condition improves.

Another interesting case began with a telephone call from a man desperate to return to work. Originally a case of acute onset back pain, the treatments he sought were not successful and the pain had become chronic over an eighteen-month period. His complaint included the original back pain and referred pain down one leg. The rearward curve in his lumbar spine seemed pronounced. His radiographer's report noted a "right-facing concavity of the lumbar spine" but normal joint structures and no disc abnormalities. When I tested this man, I found a leg-length difference of about half to three-quarters of an inch (12–15 millimeters), and a commensurate pattern of flexibility. The referred pain was experienced in the longer leg. A heel insert and just three stretching exercises had this person back at his job with much reduced discomfort. He called me recently to let me know that he was still well after a year. He said that, provided he did the exercises once or twice a week, he had no problems. In his case, I believe that the original trauma (he had slipped walking down the stairway from a local-service light plane two years previously) had resulted in a muscle injury that, due to the leg-length difference, had not had a chance to recover fully. The pain he suffered appeared to be located in the *quadratus lumborum* muscles on the side of the longer leg. Accordingly, a heel lift of three-eighths of an inch (five millimeters) and appropriate stretching exercises were prescribed. In his example, the side-bending with legs apart stretch provided immediate relief from the back pain itself, and a comparison of the *hip flexors* (muscles that lift the thigh to the chest) revealed one to be very much tighter than the other. Stretching this muscle group made a visible difference to the shape of his lower back within a couple of weeks.

Of course, not all case studies document these kinds of successes. It would be remiss of me not to mention a failure or two as well, in the interests of admitting the limits of this approach. A young woman saw me about five years ago with back pain, which her doctor had said was caused by a partial extrusion of the *nucleus pulposus*, the gelatinous core of the intervertebral disc. He advised surgery, but because her symptoms had not progressed to the stage of displaying serious neurological deficits, she felt that a conservative, exercise-based approach would be worth trying. I treated her a couple of times with shiatsu and, although we identified the exercises that gave her relief at the time and whose effects lasted a few days or so, eventually the pain became so intense that she had to have the operation. About eight months was needed for her to determine the outcome of the operation, which was successful. She continues to do the exercises from time to time, and reports that her back has much improved. Her surgeon remarked to her that her rapid recovery from the operation (she was walking around normally two weeks later) was likely due in part to the suppleness she acquired doing the exercises before the operation.

The final case study I saved until last because in one sense it is the most dramatic. A small middle-aged woman came to me complaining of "excruciating" back pain. She had not responded to any treatment and she seemed to have tried them all. Back pain had plagued her for 14 years, she said. Her job entailed travelling extensively, and she felt that the many hours she spent in the car each week were contributing to her problem. As an aside, I must note that the majority of patients know far more about their condition than most practitioners seem to give them credit for. She had bought an expensive after-market seat for her car, featuring an adjustable lumbar roll and firm side supports. The pain had not improved with this modification, but neither had it worsened over the previous year. The pain was so intense at night that her physical relationship with her husband was nonexistent. Needless to say, both were strongly affected by the illness. I began with a leg-length test which revealed a small (few millimeters) difference. Hip flexion and hamstring flexibility were within normal limits and not significantly dissimilar, I thought. When I tested her for hip flexor (*iliopsoas*) tightness, quite a different picture emerged. One hip flexor showed the normal range of movement. Coincidentally, I had begun this test sequence with this leg. After I tested the other, which was so tight that the leg would not move past the mid-line of the body before doing a Contract-Relax (C–R) stretch, she stood up next to the massage table she was using for support. She had a very peculiar look on her face—fear mixed with shock. I asked her what was wrong. She replied that this instant in time was the first time in 14 years that her back was not "killing" her. This state of affairs continues to this day, and she calls me every six months or so to let me know how she is doing.

I know that this particular example may appear to border on the incredible, perhaps even unbelievable. I could not accept it myself at the time, and months after the consultation I was sure that any day I would receive a call from her to say that her old problem had returned. I can only surmise that some fibers of the hip flexor group were extraordinarily tight and, in addition to their contribution to the extreme tension in the lumbar region, were causing the rotation of one vertebra with respect to its neighbors, and hence the pain. It is also likely that the enforced flexion of the hip joint (brought about by all those years spent in a car) may have contributed significantly to this aspect of the problem.

Posture & Flexibility at the Australian National University

When I returned from Japan and enrolled at the ANU, I decided to start an exercise class. My main motive was to ensure that I did enough stretching exercise myself each week. From one class per week in 1987, the course (named *Posture & Flexibility*) has grown to 20 classes per week in 1998. In addition, we teach another five to seven classes called *Strength & Flexibility*, where the emphasis is on accelerated strength acquisition techniques. I have taught all the teachers myself, and they come from diverse backgrounds. All attend the weekly advanced class, where information is shared and new techniques tested.

The exercise forms that have strongly influenced my present work are Yoga (hatha yoga, and more particularly the *Iyengar* style) and two traditional Japanese forms (*Makko Hoo* and *Jikyo Jutsu*).

None is complete in my opinion and I have taken liberally from all three. Where I have identified a significant lack in all three forms (for example, in specific neck exercises), I have relied on my anatomical understanding to develop an appropriate movement. Recognizing that these traditional exercise forms have objectives other than the acquisition of flexibility, I have taken from any relevant form (including dance and gymnastics) solely on the basis of furthering the goal of becoming more flexible. In this way, the goal became a *de facto* framework for relating forms which technically or historically were unrelated and whose traditional adherents (as often as not) would not like to see related. All exercises presented have been tested on thousands of patients and students.

Very early in my attempts to formulate an approach to stretching exercise, I realized that the conventional approaches to *teaching* exercise also had serious shortcomings. As mentioned earlier, of all the exercise forms I've experienced, yoga is closest to being complete in its stretching and strengthening effects but approaches to teaching it vary from insufficiently precise to doctrinaire. I also found that some of the recommendations for poses (like the lotus) made in the most reputable of textbooks are potentially dangerous, or simply wrong when considered from an anatomical perspective. Here I am not speaking of the putative effects of a pose, which often defy explanation in the scientific framework. I am talking of advice like the need to "endure excruciating pain in the knees" when practicing *padmaasana* (the lotus pose). The point here is that this kind of pain will only be felt if the hip joint has insufficient external rotation to permit the movement. My view is that a number of partial poses that foster this capacity in the hip joints should be used before attempting the pose, because it is potentially dangerous to use the knees in the strongly flexed position to generate rotational forces in the hip. This is because there is a real danger of overstretching the knee ligaments, which are maximally exposed in this position, and much of the strength of the knee in daily life derives from ligament strength.

After teaching stretching exercise for more than fifteen years, I suppose the most obvious conclusion I have reached is that age is no barrier to improvement. The older student usually progresses at a slower rate than a younger one, but the difference is nowhere as great as one might expect. I have also noticed that improvement in flexibility is slower in the initial weeks and months of a new stretching routine than are the results of a comparable amount of time spent on strength or aerobic training. However, improvement and its consequent effects are relative. Any improvement in flexibility—no matter how small in absolute terms—is experienced as a major positive event by the person concerned. Even in the most stubborn case, the absolute improvement in a particular aspect of flexibility is about 10% in a year, and the sensations of daily life are changed significantly in the person enjoying this improvement on a daily basis.

Feedback from many students over the years permits me to make some concluding remarks about the relation of practice and the outcomes of illness or injury. Students report a range of benefits. When pressed for detail, they may reply that odd random aches or pains have disappeared. Some say that movement in daily life has taken on a quality of pleasure that was not previously present. However, others have been far more specific about effects. Many people come to the classes because of the kinds of neck or back pain rife among academics and students, so that the next most commonly heard remark is that the original complaint is much improved or "cured" completely. This is also true (although to a lesser extent, admittedly) for more insidious complaints such as repetitive strain injury (RSI), or occupational overuse syndrome (OOS), where the neck, shoulder and arm exercises have proved beneficial in the majority of cases. It should be noted that in these kinds of illnesses lifestyle modification is usually required for best results. As most academics and students are unable or unwilling to do this for various reasons, the exercise classes are often used as a means of coping with the problem.

Contact address and e-mail

I am very interested in people's experiences of using the approaches detailed in the book, and this edition has benefitted from the suggestions of a great many readers. To that end, I have provided my work address for correspondence. Any suggestions or criticism will be considered and incorporated with acknowledgment in future editions.

Kit Laughlin
LPO Box 159
Australian National University
Canberra, ACT 2601
AUSTRALIA

e-mail: kit.laughlin@anu.edu.au

CHAPTER ONE

SELF-DIAGNOSIS

What is covered in this chapter?

This chapter covers our approach to self-diagnosis of neck and back pain, and is based on the process we use in the *Overcome neck & back pain* workshops. This approach is most suitable for people who suspect that their neck or back pain is largely muscular in origin. Please read through the entire test procedure, have a quick look at the exercises mentioned, and when you are ready to do the tests put aside an hour or so where you will not be disturbed. Page 28 shows a sample self-assessment of the type we use in the workshops—photocopy and use it. Take your time, and write down what you find—the results of the various exercises we use as tests will give you your exercise plan. A simplified flow chart of the testing procedure for muscular imbalances will be found towards the end of this chapter, but do not rely on it alone.

This approach assumes that you are not suffering neurological deficits, a term that describes symptoms like: back pain that hurts as much at night as during the day, unrelenting pain down the back of the leg, areas of numbness on the buttocks or on the legs or feet, pins and needles in the feet, wasting of the leg muscles, or loss of feeling in part of the legs or feet. Similar signs may be present in the arms or hands. These are symptoms that require the attention of a specialist. If you have good and bad days, though, or your sciatica is intermittent, you may proceed with the following tests, but be careful. This chapter is not intended as a substitute for professional medical care, and as I mentioned in the *Cautions* section in the preface, you should consult with your regular health care professional before embarking on the particular exercises that the self-diagnosis will indicate. You may have a specific condition that could be worsened by using certain exercises—check to be sure.

The self-diagnosis involves three main aspects: i) **determination of whether you have one hip lower than the other** when standing or sitting (*pelvic obliquity*, in medical terminology, and which may affect back or neck problems), **ii) determination of whether muscular causes of problems like *sciatica* are present**, and **iii) determination of your pattern of muscular tension**, regardless of whether other causes may be present. The neck exercises follow the back exercises, but even if you are only concerned with neck problems, the best results will be experienced by doing the back assessment and exercises first. If you wish, however, you may turn to the neck exercises directly after reading the introduction to chapter two if you feel that you have no need of the back assessment. Exercises 15 to 21 cover the neck region, and exercise 12 stretches the middle of the back.

In chapter one I wish to present only the practical methods we use in the workshops, so you can get to the right exercises as soon as possible. Chapter four, "The causes of neck and back pain," goes into more technical and medical detail. The order of the exercises we use in the workshops is a little different from the order of the book, because the workshops assume that the participants have immediate problems (and where a specific order through the exercises is indicated for safety and other reasons) whereas the book is arranged roughly from the easiest exercises to the most difficult. **If you do not have immediate problems, you may skip this chapter and go to chapter two.** If you are interested in trying to diagnose your problem in the terms described, especially if yours is a recurring problem, read on.

Pelvic obliquity

We have found that a tilting of the hips to one side is the most common contributing cause of recurring middle and low back pain, and it may be a contributing cause of neck pain. Plato wrote about leg-length differences and their relation to back problems two and a half thousand years ago, so the idea is hardly new. The problem is that most people assume that they are symmetrical. You should know that over half the population have an actual leg-length difference, ranging from just under a quarter of an inch up to three-quarters of an inch (or more) in the length of their leg bones. This has been determined by a number of studies using whole-body X-rays. The question of whether small differences can be significant is explored in chapter four, and the studies dealing with leg-length inequality (with precise measurements) will be found there too.

We have found that these sorts of differences are a major contributing cause of back pain, and have come to this conclusion for three main reasons. If you do have such a difference, your patterns of flexibility can be predicted with a good degree of reliability, and we assume that this is not coincidental. This aspect will be addressed later, so you can use this as a check on the leg-length test result. Another reason is that we have found quite characteristic differences in the shape and size of the lumbar and middle back muscles related to tilted hips, and you may well be able to see this for yourself, when you know where to look. The last reason is that a great many people have gained significant relief from their neck or back pain by only correcting part of an identified difference, even if they do not do the recommended exercises. It is also true that there are people who have demonstrable leg-length differences and who have no neck or back problems—one of my exercise teachers has a leg-length difference of just under an inch, with no problems, but he also has superior strength and flexibility. If you have neck or back problems, especially of a recurring nature, and a leg-length difference, I suggest strongly that it be identified and corrected.

How to determine if you have one hip lower than the other

We use a standing test to determine pelvic obliquity. I use this rather technical term, because there are a number of causes of one hip being lower than the other, and not all are related to leg-length. I go into these other causes in chapter four; all we want to know at this point is whether you display this condition yourself. I should note here that you may have been told already that you have a "short leg," following the use of a different procedure. I suggest strongly that you repeat the tests as described below, because we have found that the standard tests done in the lying position can give false results, and even whole body radiographs ("X-rays") can be misleading. The human eye, however, is very effective at picking difference, and in the test we use any significant difference will be visible. We will examine the whole body from the feet to the upper back, and the observations used to gain an insight to how your body uses itself, and why.

To begin the tests, you will need a partner to look at you and a book or piece of wood around half an inch in thickness. Try to find a room where the light comes through a window. Preferably, you stand naked in front of your partner, facing away from them, and with the light shining *across your body*. Standing this way will reveal the contours of the back muscles. The reason for doing the test naked is to avoid the distraction of the horizontal lines that clothes impose on the shape of your body, but if this suggestion is impractical, wear tight exercise-type shorts or leggings—any clothing where the shape of the body is visible. We need to see the skin and muscles of the lower and middle back. We would like to be able to see the fold between the bottom and the legs (the *gluteal fold*), too, as it is a useful landmark. If you do not have a partner, the tests can be done on your own, but it is harder to see what we are looking for when you look at the body from the front. Nonetheless, it can be done, and I will describe this below.

Stand as suggested, with your weight evenly on both feet, *and the inside edges of your feet parallel.* This is essential, because if you do have a difference, one of the ways you compensate is by standing with more of your weight on the shorter leg and with its foot pointing roughly straight ahead. The other leg will be turned more out to the side, and with less weight on it. These are generalizations; what I mean is that (for example) in the course of an evening standing around at a party, you will tend to stand as described more often than another way. Chapter four explores the reasons why—here, it is enough to say that if you want reliable results from the test, stand with weight evenly on both feet, and both feet parallel. This feels quite strange for some people.

The following directions are for your partner. Look at his or her feet: are the ankles (specifically, the *Achilles tendon*) straight, or do they roll inwards (*pronation*). Unless the ankles are visibly pronated, there is probably no significance for back problems. (If you do have pronating ankles, consider seeing a *podiatrist*; these practitioners specialize in *orthotics*, devices that fit into the shoe to stabilize the position of the foot in relation to the leg.) If they both look the same, look at the calf muscles next: they should look the same, too. If one appears larger than the other, note it. We have found that in the majority of people, the larger calf muscle is found on the shorter leg, but some people use other compensation mechanisms, so don't jump to conclusions.

Now stand well back from the person you are examining, and look at the whole body. What we would like to see, but rarely do, is a straight spine when viewed from behind. Additionally, we would like to see symmetrical development of the lower and middle back muscles, the large ones that run up and down both sides of the spine. Does one side of the pair look thicker, or wider—in other words, better developed? We have found that the majority of people with pelvic obliquity show better development of the lumbar muscles on the short-leg side, but again, don't jump to conclusions; just note what you see. Pay attention to the line of the bottom; are the gluteal folds horizontal, and the same on both sides? Then look at the hip bones (the *iliac crests*)—these should be horizontal. If you are looking at a woman, are the dimples at the back of the hips level? (The dimples are 3–4 inches below the pant waistline.) When you look at the lower back, is it straight (vertical) and symmetrical when compared with the hips? Are there any sideways curves?

Now look at the middle back: does the spine of the middle back look straight from behind? Is it directly in line with the lumbar spine? Take a look now at the whole of the middle and lower back, and see if you can see any sort of misalignment. I have deliberately not mentioned the level of the shoulders to this point, even though this was probably one of the things you noticed on first looking. This is because a number of factors can contribute to uneven shoulders, and some of these are not related to lower and middle back problems—concentrate on looking at the lower half of the body first. In men, the most reliable indicators of difference are the lumbar muscles; in women, look to see if one hip seems fuller, or more rounded, than the other, and at the levelness of the dimples at the back of the hips. One hip can seem fuller if it is more to one side of the center of the body than the other. If your partner is naked, the *gluteal folds* are useful markers, as I mentioned. The folds of fat above the waist (the "love handles") are not particularly good landmarks, we've found; fat distribution may not be symmetrical at all.

Now examine the first photograph, showing me from behind, standing with my weight evenly on both feet. If you are like most people, you will find it difficult to be certain about any difference you can see in the first photograph. For most people not trained to look at the body in this "global" way, your partner will look much the same in their right and left halves; that is, nothing much will stand out. Now we bring out the book or the piece of wood I mentioned before. If you suspect that one hip is lower than the other, put the block under the *longer* leg first; ask your partner to again stand with weight on both legs equally (both feet still pointing straight ahead) and step back and look again, going through all the points of the last paragraphs, concentrating on hips, lower and middle back. Now remove the block, and place it under the other leg, check weight distribution and foot placement, and look at the hip and lower back region once again. Three results are possible:

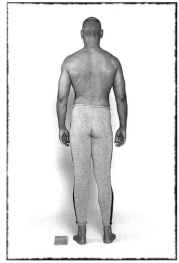

i) one hip is lifted higher than the other

The most common finding is that the block seems to distort the shape of the spine and the level of the hips much more when it is placed under one foot than the other. This suggests that either one leg is actually shorter than the other, or that one ankle is strongly pronating while the other does not (but you will have noted this already, in your examination of the feet), that the femur neck angles are different left to right, that the hip joints are placed unequally in the pelvis (very unlikely, but still possible) or that one half of the pelvis is smaller that the other (a condition called *small hemipelvis*). A seated test described in chapter four will identify these last two causes, if there are significant differences. (In the workshops run in 1996–1997, where we examined around 1,500 people, we found this condition spectacularly exhibited in about thirty-five people.) An actual leg-length difference is the most common explanation for the results described.

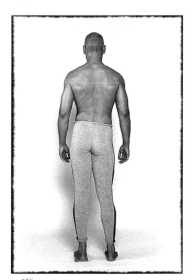

Look at the second photograph to help you—can you see how distorted my body has become? Here, the block is placed under my longer leg, and the body symmetry is clearly changed: the lateral curves in the spine are accentuated, one hip is obviously higher that the other, the back muscles on the lower-hip side stand out more. Look at the final photograph for comparison: now the block is under the shorter leg, and the whole body looks far more symmetrical. The block I am standing on is just over half an inch in thickness.

Now ask your partner how she or he feels about the block under each foot. The most common response is that the block feels better under one foot, and that this will coincide with your observations of hip levelness. Be aware, though, that a small percentage of people will say that the block feels better under the leg which seems the longer to you, as the observer. What can this mean? The most common reason is that placing

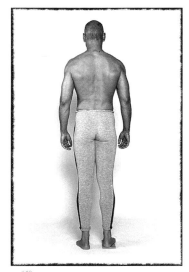

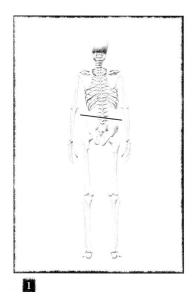

1

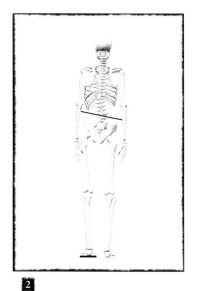

2

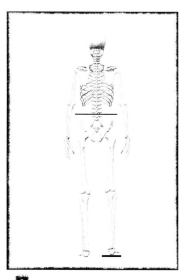

3

the block under one leg relieves pressure from a structure on the back or in the hip that is currently inflamed or pressure-sensitive; we have found this result in people with *sacro-iliac joint* problems most commonly. I suggest retesting these people after doing the exercises indicated by the functional tests described below. Usually, after doing the right exercises, the sensations your partner will report from the leg length test will coincide with your observations.

A further possibility is that your partner *feels no difference* one side to the other, even though the difference is obvious to an observer. This indicates how far the body will compensate itself to feel balanced. Say nothing—but repeat the test from side to side, letting the person stand on the block for half a minute on each side. We have never had to repeat this procedure more than two or three times before the person being tested suddenly becomes aware that the block feels much worse (or less often, much better) under one heel. Note your partner's reactions, and check them against the tests of functional flexibility described below.

ii) both hips are lifted by the test, but one higher than the other

Supposing, though, that the block you chose to use in the test lifted both hips up from level, but seemed to lift one higher than the other—what might this mean? This second possible test result suggests that there is a difference, but that the block you are using is too thick. Use a block of around half the thickness, or if you are using a book, open it halfway, and repeat the test. If you have selected the right thickness (that is, roughly equal to the leg-length difference) then the support will seem to elevate only one hip; this is the longer leg. When the same thickness is placed under the shorter leg, everything looks about right. Note the thickness of the support. On the workshops, we use quarter-inch and half-inch blocks only for this test. Again, after you have tested your partner with the smaller support, ask him or her to report the sensations; again, the most common response is to agree with what you find; that is, they will most often say that the support feels better under the foot of what you believe to be the shorter leg.

iii) both hips are lifted about the same

The third possible result is that the block distorts the shape of the spine and the level of the hips equally on both sides. If this is your observation, now ask your partner what he or she feels, with the block placed under each foot in turn. Most people will report sensations that will coincide with your impressions; that is, if you see the same degree of distortion produced by the block on both sides, they are most likely to say that the block feels equally uncomfortable (or equally comfortable) under each foot. When your observation of no significant difference coincides with the reported sensations, conclude no significant difference, and move on to the Tests of muscular imbalance, below. Occasionally, however, someone will say that the block feels more comfortable under one foot than the other, but to you the observer the block seems to change the alignment and shape of the spine equally. Note this observation, do the exercise tests, and redo the standing leg-length test. For the majority that we've tested, people report that the block now feels about the same under either foot.

The heel insert

If you find a difference and your partner agrees with you, what do you do? We have found that the use of an insert of a particular thickness, made from a relatively incompressible material and placed in the heel of the shorter leg, usually gives results that are noticeable within a week or so. Look at the illustration: the insert should be nontapering, from three to four inches in length (depending on the size of your foot), and the front half-inch should be tapered as shown, to avoid irritating the bottom of the foot. Leather is an excellent material for inserts, and there are half-a-dozen proprietary closed-cell foam equivalents, available from podiatrists, chiropractors and osteopaths, or your local shoemaker. To be sure of the test results try an insert made out of cardboard or a similar material for a few weeks to see if there is any determinable difference in the way your back feels, before spending money.

How thick should the insert be?

For reasons I go into in chapter four, I have found that an insert of a thickness *something less than half* any identified difference is the best place to start. We use quarter-inch and half-inch blocks to test leg-length difference in the workshops, starting the test with the thicker of the two. If this turns out to be too thick (both hips lifted, but one more that the other) we re-test using the smaller block. So, if you need the thicker block to make you level, we would recommend an insert of around a quarter of an inch, or a bit less, around three-sixteenths. And if the smaller block seems better, then we would recommend an insert of around an eighth of an inch. We have found that it is better to be conservative in the choice of correction thickness first up; you can always increase the thickness as your body gets used

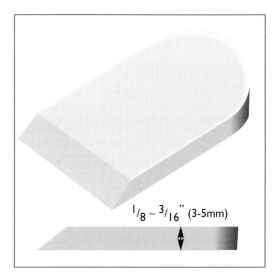

Heel insert

to it. Too thick an insert and you may give yourself other problems—remember your body has spent years getting used to its difference, and we don't want to interfere with the body's adaptation mechanisms too directly.

What if I make a mistake?

What if your partner has made a mistake and has told you that your right leg seems shorter but in fact it is the left—what can happen then? We have found a few people who have been told that one leg is shorter than the other, and an insert prescribed, and in the workshops we have found that in fact it is the other shoe that needed the insert. Sometimes, the initial determination was made on the basis of a *lying* leg-length test. I have not found these tests to be consistently reliable, and I will explain why in chapter four. No matter how the original testing was done, I recommend strongly that the test be repeated in the standing, load-bearing position, as described. Normally, we have found that if someone has been wrongly advised, and uses an insert incorrectly, their condition worsens. If the correct leg has been identified and an appropriate insert used, the vast majority find that improvement is immediate, and that they feel more balanced in walking. If you have been told that you *do* have a leg-length difference, but that it is insignificant, please do the test described anyway: we have found that, depending on the lifestyle and activities of the individual, leg-length differences of one-eighth of an inch can be significant. If both you and the partner testing you find a difference one side to the other, the difference is likely to be significant. What have you got to lose? Try the recommended insert and the worst that can happen is your condition will be slightly worsened, or not affected. If this occurs, discard the insert. The best that can happen is that the condition improves significantly.

Other indicators of pelvic obliquity

I have left these minor indicators to last, as I have found the standing test to be the most reliable and repeatable. However, these indicators can be assessed easily, and together may provide some confirming evidence. A single indicator suggesting leg-length difference should not be taken too seriously. If the indicators together do not present a coherent picture, please repeat the standing test carefully—a single indicator can be the result of asymmetrical patterns of either strength or flexibility alone, with no pelvic obliquity.

Lie down face up with the legs together, and settle yourself. Look down your body and check to see if you are aligned correctly; that is, the body and the legs are a straight line. Close your eyes, lightly press the toes together, and relax completely, letting the feet fall apart to the outside. Now lift your head and look at your feet (or ask your partner to look for you) and try to see whether one foot falls further to the outside. We have found in the majority of people with demonstrated leg-length difference that *the longer leg falls further outside* (technically speaking, external hip rotation is greater on the long leg side).

The next test requires two kitchen scales. I suggest calibrating the scales; do this by placing an object on one of the scales and noting the reading. Place the same object on the second scale, and adjust it so that it reads the same as the first one. Place them side by side, with a couple of inches in between. Stand on the scales. Again close your eyes (this is to deactivate the standard balance feedback mechanisms), and stand normally. Relax, open your eyes, and look down at the scales. Both should read close to the same. We have found that the majority of people with demonstrated leg-length difference rest *more weight on the shorter leg*. Note the results.

Next, find an old pair of shoes; if you are a runner or jogger, or walk recreationally, the shoes you wear for these activities will be ideal. If you work on your feet all day, check those shoes or boots. Tennis and squash players need to be careful in interpreting the wear patterns on their playing shoes, because the serving action causes its own patterns, frequently overlying and confusing any basic gait-related patterns that may be there. Walking shoes would be better to use as the indicator in this case. If your gait is even (common in symmetrical people) we find that the wear patterns are close to identical. The most common pattern (but a rather smaller majority than the other indicators) is that the shoe of the shorter leg is more worn, but the pattern depends crucially on what your body has decided is *its normal leg*. By this I mean that some people's bodies regard the long leg as normal, and tend to "fall" down slightly onto the shorter leg. This is the more common pattern. But some people's bodies regard the short leg as normal, and "climb" onto the longer leg, wearing this shoe more. From the shoe pattern alone, I feel that you cannot infer anything useful, except that *if there is a difference in wear pattern, it needs to be explained*. One of my patients, for example, complained of one-sided lower back pain, and displayed the one-sided lower back muscle development characteristic of an actual leg-length difference, with her right calf muscle noticeably better developed that the left. Jumping to conclusions (something I warn my students about continuously), I performed the standing leg-length test—and no difference was the result. This was confusing—and I asked her what her hobbies were. She told me she was a "pro-am" (professional-amateur) Highland dancer—and one of the signature elements of that form of dance is multiple turns done on the ball of the foot of the right leg! Moral of the story? Be careful in assessment and don't jump to conclusions!

The last one I have saved to the end, because it is mainly anecdotal. When we have identified leg-length difference, so many people have looked at me quizzically, and asked whether this might not have something to do with the fact that they have had to take up the hem of skirts (or the cuffs of trousers) more on one side than the other their whole lives. The answer is yes, of course, and I want to remind you of a truism we have discovered in the vast majority of people: we all think that we are symmetrical; accordingly that is what we see. Try to see what is really there. Remember, "normal" for each individual, and "desirable" are completely different notions, and we all get used to how we are.

How to determine whether muscular causes of problems like sciatica are present

A note about how to use the self-assessment sheet. Note that the exercise numbers are in the left-hand column. As you go through the exercises, it is essential to record the tighter or more painful side of those exercises that permit comparison of left and right, to note the version you used (which always should be the **easiest** one to begin with), and in the "Reaction" column, note your feelings on doing the exercise. Here are the sorts of reactions you might note: did it make the problem feel better? Worse? Not much effect? The next time you go through the list, these notes will alert you to any special consideration required. And if an exercise didn't affect you particularly (I assume here that you did it properly) you may leave it out of your routine, trying it again in a few weeks' time. In this way, we will arrive at a short, efficient list of your own exercises, *to be done twice a week only*, in the beginning. Also note the exercises you may have needed to repeat, in order that the back felt more comfortable at the end of the session.

We begin with these exercises in order to determine whether certain muscles in the hip are causing the variety of problems referred to with this term. Literally, "sciatica" means pain in the sciatic nerve, but general use can also mean pain down the back of the leg or pain in the hip. I go into the possible causes of this problem in chapter four. We have found that a muscle in the hip called *piriformis* can give rise to the majority of symptoms that are usually associated with impingement of the sciatic nerve by extruding disk material or the structures of the spine itself. We have found that the standard diagnostic tests are not reliable in distinguishing these different causes, so we recommend trying one of the *piriformis* stretches to see whether there is any benefit to be gained. To make the test more objective, I suggest having your partner help you do a *hamstring* muscle stretch, in the lying face-up position, **exercise 11.** Try to get an idea of how far the leg will come off the floor. **Partner: be extremely gentle, moving the leg very slowly into the stretch position.** The reasons for this caution are expanded in chapter four. Also, note any left/right differences.

A number of results are possible. If you found that having your leg stretched in the exercise 11 position gave you pain in your back (rather than a stretch being felt in your hip, leg or calf muscle) note this down, and we will return to it below. This result could indicate that nerve impingement is present. **Do the following three additional exercise tests very carefully** (both C–Rs of exercise 11, exercise 30, and exercise 6), and note the results. It is not uncommon for the test results of exercise 11 to improve after doing these exercises, even when there is evidence of disc or vertebral structure impingement, as the possible muscular causes identified may be adding to the problem.

If you feel *pain in the calf muscle* as the leg reaches the stretch position, get off the floor and do **exercise 30.** Although found in the Prevention section, you may try this exercise, with the Contract–Relax (C–R) component (for a fuller description, see the relevant section in chapter two). Again have your partner stretch the leg in the lying face-up position described in exercise 11. If the leg goes higher on the second stretch, note down "tight calf muscles," and include exercise 30 in your list of necessary exercises. Note any left/right differences in tightness in the calf muscles.

If you felt *the main effects in the back of the thigh*, somewhere between the buttock and the knee, but no pain in the back, have your partner help you with the two C–R stretches found in exercise 11. If the leg goes higher after doing these two stretches than previously, suspect that you have tight hamstrings , and add exercise 11 to your list. Note any right/left differences in the hamstring muscles.

If stretching the leg in exercise 11 caused pain in the buttock of the leg being stretched, and you *felt this stretch or pain sensation down the back of the thigh* of the same leg, go to the first of the *piriformis* stretches, **exercise 6.** Note any differences in stretching sensation or flexibility in the exercise. After doing exercise 6 and concentrating on the C–R part, again have your partner do the lying face-up stretch in exercise 11. If your leg goes higher after doing exercise 6, suspect that *piriformis* might be involved in your problem, and try **exercise 7** also. Retest with exercise 11.

How to determine your patterns of muscular tension

Now it is time to start the left/right comparison of trunk function. We begin our tests of functional flexibility with **exercise 5,** which will give us an insight into hip joint tightness, and give us an idea whether the *hip flexors* (muscles at the front of the hip) are involved in your problem. Read all the directions for exercise 5 carefully, do the exercise and note where you feel the main effects. If you *feel the effects mainly in the buttock muscles* (and perhaps part of the *hamstring* muscles (the muscles at the back of thigh), then add **exercises 5 and 11** to your list of necessary exercises, and your choice of the *piriformis* stretches, **exercises 6, 7 or 8**. On the other hand, if most of the stretch effect was *felt in the front of the back leg*, suspect tight hip flexors, and add **exercises 9 and 27** (the latter for the *quadriceps*, the large front thigh muscles) to your list. Be aware that when doing exercise 5 as a test, you may find the hip is tight when one foot is placed to the front, but the hip flexors tight when the other foot is placed to the front. This kind of asymmetry is common, and we believe it to be a major cause of back problems. *Note any right/left differences.* We will be doing twice the amount of work for the tight side of any pair of muscles where we find this kind of difference, so you need to know your own pattern.

Next we turn to **exercises 1 and 2,** which I have grouped for convenience because both involve bending forwards in a supported way, using a chair. Take care to note which side seems tighter or more painful in exercise 2 (here, we need to know which is the tighter of the sides you are bending *away* from). The tighter or more painful side in this movement will usually test similar in **exercise 3** (the solo version of exercise 4), **exercise 4,** and **exercise 10.** In addition, exercises 1 and 2 are excellent gentle warming-up movements for later stretches.

Now read the directions for **exercise 4,** and ask your partner to help. Note any differences left to right, especially if rotating in one direction seems to elicit pain similar to your back pain. We have found that doing the exercise in the suggested way can make a sore back feel immediately better. Again, note down whether moving to one side is either more restricted or more painful than the other—these differences become your exercise plan.

Next we move to what we have found to be the major lower back exercise, offered in two basic versions. Only do the version you can; read the directions of **exercise 10** carefully. We have found that bending the trunk to the side in the manner described (either the chair or the floor version) seems to provide the fastest relief of most lower back pain. Take your time trying these movements: they are strong exercises, and you will need to be careful.

You finish the test session with whichever of the exercises made your back most comfortable. Most people find **exercise 3 or 4, or 1 and 2** have a pleasing effect. If you are a *sciatica* sufferer, though, it might be that one of the *piriformis* exercises (**6, 7 or 8**) will be the best one to finish on.

I said above that I would come back to those people whose backs felt sore on doing the hamstring test above, **exercise 11.** This result, especially if unchanged after doing the calf muscle stretch (**exercise 30**), the two C–R stretches from **exercise 11,** and the *piriformis* stretches (**exercises 6, 7 and 8**) suggests that there may be nerve impingement by disc material (as with a prolapsed disc) or by the structures of the spine itself. Please discuss this result with your health care professional. We have found that forward bending (**exercises 1 and 2,** the rotation movements (**exercises 3 and 4**) and the side-bending movements (**exercises 2 and 10**) can be very effective, especially bending away from the side of the prolapse. Please note that bending *towards* the side of a disc prolapse may reproduce impingement symptoms in the feet or legs; if so, do the exercise on this side very gently. Bending *away* from the affected side immediately after will settle these symptoms down.

For people with neck problems, please note that pelvic obliquity can have a significant effect here, too. I go into the question of how a leg-length difference is resolved at the neck level later, because this aspect may be complicated by dominant arm considerations. For now, if there is a difference, experiment with the correction as suggested.

If **middle back** pain is your major concern, test yourself with **exercise 12**. If this helps, look carefully at **exercise 14**. This is a difficult exercise for some people for physical proportion reasons, but together with exercise 12 is very effective for these problems.

There is no special way of going through the neck exercises—we have found the presented order effective, so follow **exercises 15 to 21 as they are presented**, again noting any left/right differences. Assess each exercise by itself, and don't assume that if you are tight on the right-hand side in exercise 17, for example, that you will be tight on the same side in exercise 20. Try them all, and note the results.

Now look at your sheet: it is a blueprint for your own exercise program, to be followed *twice a week* for four to eight weeks before reassessment. You don't need to do all the exercises listed: choose the ones which seemed to be the most effective. Four or five exercises should be sufficient in the first few weeks. Please begin each exercise by *doing the side that was tighter* (or more painful) in the assessment first, doing the exercise for the other, less problematic side, *and repeating the exercise for the first side.* In this way, your problem parts will get twice the work of the rest of your body, and will adapt the fastest. In time, both sides of the body will feel and function remarkably similarly. Add additional exercises as your body loosens, and retest yourself using all the exercises listed every month or so.

The final word in this section relating to leg-length inequality may be stated now. We have found that there is a predictable pattern to this asymmetry, which you may check against your exercise test results. Here is the pattern:

Assuming that the right leg is the shorter, the hip muscles (as tested in the first part of exercise 3) will test *looser* on the right leg.

Less reliable, but still prevalent in the majority, the right-leg side will test *looser* in the rotation part of exercise 3 when it is taken towards the floor.

The hamstring muscles are *looser* on the short-leg side (exercise 11).

The *hip flexors* will be *tighter* on the short-leg side (exercise 9).

Bending away from the short-leg side is *tighter* in lateral flexion (exercise 10).

How does your pattern look in comparison? I must stress that these patterns are not absolute; the most reliable ones are exercises 3 (hip stretch) and 11; and the least reliable is the hip flexor relation (exercise 9), but the pattern described is the one we have found to be most commonly presented after testing thousands of people, and one of the reasons I believe that even small leg-length differences can be significant.

FLOW CHART FOR TESTING MUSCLE IMBALANCES

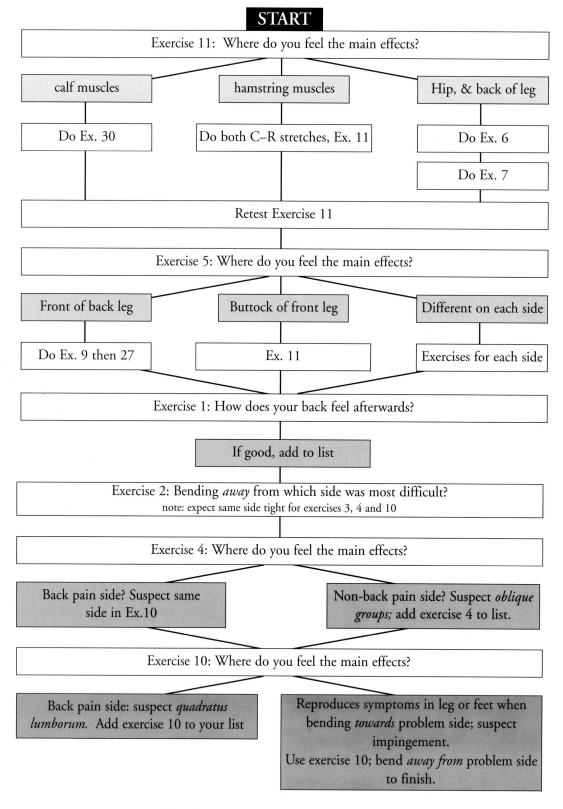

START

Exercise 11: Where do you feel the main effects?

calf muscles	hamstring muscles	Hip, & back of leg
Do Ex. 30	Do both C–R stretches, Ex. 11	Do Ex. 6
		Do Ex. 7

Retest Exercise 11

Exercise 5: Where do you feel the main effects?

Front of back leg	Buttock of front leg	Different on each side
Do Ex. 9 then 27	Ex. 11	Exercises for each side

Exercise 1: How does your back feel afterwards?

If good, add to list

Exercise 2: Bending *away* from which side was most difficult?
note: expect same side tight for exercises 3, 4 and 10

Exercise 4: Where do you feel the main effects?

Back pain side? Suspect same side in Ex.10	Non-back pain side? Suspect *oblique groups;* add exercise 4 to list.

Exercise 10: Where do you feel the main effects?

Back pain side: suspect *quadratus lumborum.* Add exercise 10 to your list	Reproduces symptoms in leg or feet when bending *towards* problem side; suspect impingement. Use exercise 10; bend *away from* problem side to finish.

Finish with whichever exercise made your back feel best.

Where am I sore?

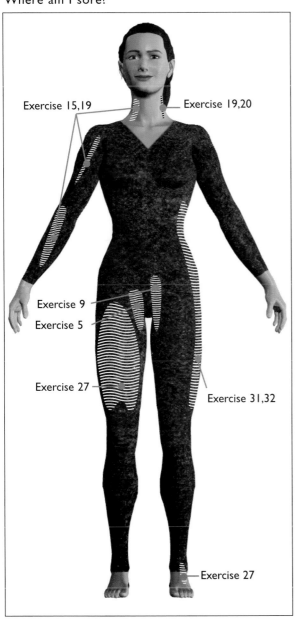

Exercise 15,19

Exercise 19,20

Exercise 9

Exercise 5

Exercise 27

Exercise 31,32

Exercise 27

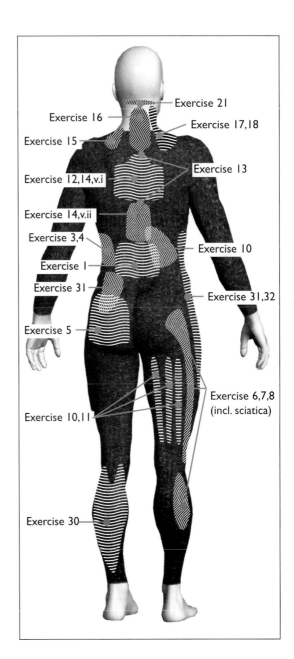

Exercise 16

Exercise 21

Exercise 15

Exercise 17,18

Exercise 12,14,v.i

Exercise 13

Exercise 14,v.ii

Exercise 3,4

Exercise 10

Exercise 1

Exercise 31

Exercise 31,32

Exercise 5

Exercise 10,11

Exercise 6,7,8
(incl. sciatica)

Exercise 30

Note: only one muscle of each matched pair is shown, for simplicity

TEST AND EXERCISE CHECK LIST

Standing leg-length test:

With block, one hip elevated; under other foot hips seem level? Suspect difference
With block, both hips lifted, but one more than the other? Try smaller block
With block, both hips lifted about the same? Suspect no significant difference

Did you find a leg-length difference? Circle:		yes	no
If yes, which leg is shorter?		left	right
If yes, big or small block?		big	small

Following the muscle imbalance flow chart, circle left or right to indicate your tight side: **Your exercise program is to be done twice per week only for the first month.** Monitor the effects, and *have an extra day off* if you need to. Exercising in the afternoon or evening is best, and have a bath to heat up the body before commencing.

Exercise	Version	Side		Reaction
Lower back exercises				
Exercise 11		left	right	
Exercise 30		left	right (optional)	
Exercise 5		left	right	
		front back	**front back**	
Exercise 6		left	right (optional)	
Exercise 7		left	right (optional)	
Exercise 8		left	right (optional)	
Exercise 9		left	right	
Exercise 27		left	right (optional)	
Exercise 1				
Exercise 2		left	right	
Exercise 3 (if on your own)		left	right	
Exercise 4		left	right	
Exercise 10		left	right	
Middle back exercises				
Exercise 12		left	right	
Exercise 14		left	right (optional)	
Neck exercises				
Exercise 15		left	right	
Exercise 16				
Exercise 17		left	right	
Exercise 18		left	right	
Exercise 19		left	right (optional)	
Exercise 20		left	right	
Exercise 21		left	right	

Test your pattern of flexibility against the pattern described at the end of chapter one.

How often should I stretch?

After you have gone through the recommended exercises and made a list of the ones that seem the most important to you, how often, and how many times, should one do the stretches described in this and the next chapter? As a general rule, do them **no less than twice a week, and no more than three times a week**, but these recommendations need some qualification.

When teaching yoga and stretching in Japan and attending intensive martial arts classes, I had the opport}nity to test the often-voiced claim that stretching needs to be done daily to be effective. Concentrating on the major *quadriceps* and *hamstring hamstrings* muscle groups, I had students working out every day, others every second day, others every third day, and others still who stretched only once a week. To my surprise, the once-every-three-days group made noticeably faster progress over six months than the other groups. The next best group was the once-a-week group, and the other two groups (every day and every second day) made similar progress. The experimental groups were people of varying ages, from teenagers to fifty-year-olds. Over time it became obvious that stretching exercise is simply another stress as far as the body is concerned, and it needs time to recover from that stress. The every-day groups often told me that when they tried to stretch the same muscles the next day, they were sore—a strong disincentive. As time went on, the every-day group made adjustments to *how* they stretched, and after a while I found that they stretched hard only once or twice per week, and stretched lightly on the other days. Because the groups that stretched less frequently made better progress, and because we are interested in an efficient and safe approach which is least likely to have adverse effects, we recommend stretching two or three times a week only.

The claim that people need to stretch every day is often made, but the reasons are not usually made clear, and confusion can be the result. For example, yoga teachers recommend daily practice because one aspect of the poses is devotional. The *asanas* are based in Indian mythology and have practical and symbolic lessons for the practitioner. Doing the poses with these ideas in mind, coupled with particular ways of breathing, helps the mind focus on these lessons. The goal of yoga is enlightenment, and daily practice is recommended. Because of this goal, in an important sense the increased flexibility of the yoga practitioner is a by-product of the practice rather than its main focus. Sophisticated selections from the wide range of available poses means that even if practice is done daily, different muscle groups are being worked on subsequent days, so the problems I mentioned earlier are avoided.

In dance and gymnastics, daily practice of stretching exercise is also recommended, although for different reasons. However, these disciplines distinguish between limber classes, which loosen up the body in preparation for the day's skill classes, and stretching, which is designed to increase the range of movement. In practice, these distinctions are often blurred and the individual concerned decides which of these goals will be pursued on any given day on an *ad hoc* basis according to how he or she feels.

Your goals can be stated clearly. You are trying to reduce your neck or back pain, and we are assuming that the right stretching exercises will help. Once you have chosen the exercises, how often should they be done? We need to tread a fine line between doing enough to have the desired effect, but not so much that you further irritate the parts of the body concerned. Every second day is the right frequency to begin with, while being prepared to modify this as you monitor the effects of the exercise. If, for example, you do the chair exercise (the first one in this chapter) and experience some relief, repeat it after a moment or two to see if a little extra movement can be achieved (and to feel the slight improvement that one almost always feels doing an exercise a second time). Do any other exercises you have chosen (once or twice), and do no more that day. When you get up the next day, see how you feel. Do no exercise on this day, but use it to monitor the effects of the previous day's exercise. Do not be surprised to feel a little muscular soreness in the places you have stretched—this is normal. Usually, muscular soreness resulting from unaccustomed stretching is quite different to the pain of the original complaint, and a sign that useful change is occurring.

On the following day, monitor the body once more, and decide whether you want to have an additional rest day (two in all) or whether you wish to try the exercises again, cautiously. Only you can decide, and often it will not be until you try the exercises that you will be able to decide. If muscular soreness is experienced, wait another day. Remember to err on the side of caution—in the beginning it is better to do too little rather than too much. The rule of thumb is, the more serious your problem, the *less* you should do. Give your body time to adjust to this new stress. In general, the rehabilitation neck exercises can be done more frequently than the back exercises. This is more to do with the size of the muscles involved than anything else (sore small muscles seem to be less of a problem than sore large ones). Ultimately, you must judge how often to do the exercises.

Let us say that a couple of months have elapsed, and the problem seems to have improved. Now you feel ready to tackle some of the more difficult prevention exercises found in chapter three. Again, it is better to do too little rather than too much. It is extremely tempting to do more, because the exercises seem to be having the effect you want, but here again you will need to restrain yourself. The exercises in chapter three are generally stronger than those in chapter two, and you will need longer recovery periods to accustom yourself to their effects in the beginning. At least one rest day (and preferably two) is recommended, although if muscular soreness persists, have an extra day or two. As before, each exercise may be done twice in any stretching session.

Finally, I wish to introduce some ideas that at first may seem to contradict the previous paragraphs. Presuming that you have been able to use the rehabilitation exercises successfully, many people find that they wish to do one or two of them more regularly than what I have suggested. Is this all right? Yes, once the original problem has settled down significantly. However, in recommending this, I wish to raise a distinction I made above (between limber and stretching workouts), but with a different slant.

Dancers and gymnasts do limber workouts to regain the flexibility of the day before, their *normal* flexibility. Activities that would look like serious stretching for most people are part of the normal vocabulary of movement for dancers and gymnasts, and are nothing more than extended warm-ups, as preparation for difficult strength or flexibility moves in the day's training. Anyone can use particular exercises to set themselves up for the day's activities in a similar way, too. Some of my students and patients use a number of the exercises on a daily basis before they go to work. If you are a morning person and feel happy with exercise done this way, there is unlikely to be a problem. Stretching exercise ideally should be done *after* you warm up, so if you walk, jog, or ride a bike, do your stretches when you return home. They are an excellent way to "warm down." However, most people are somewhat stiff in the mornings, and somewhat less sensitive to their body's feelings. If your back or neck problem is really painful, I strongly recommend that the exercises be done in the evening. Once the problem has settled down, you can revise your stretching schedule to suit.

Many students have listened to me talk about recommended frequencies of stretching, and have later said that they do some exercises every day, just because they feel good to do. I support this use wholeheartedly—but, if used in this fashion, do not try to increase the range of movement in any of the exercises every day. Rather, use them to take tension away from a particular problem area, or to try to prevent a problem from occurring, or simply to loosen yourself up. Any of the exercises may be used at the end of a day in the same way to reduce the tension acquired by the body through daily life. Again, though, distinguish between doing an exercise gently (to reduce tension and regain yesterday's looseness) and a stretching workout where you are trying to improve the range of movement of some part of the body. The latter workout will result in some muscle soreness and will require a couple of days for recovery. In fact, the dancers I have known well over the years have told me that they would do a "serious" stretch for any of their tight bits only once or twice a week—the other times they simply loosen up. You will find practical advice about breathing, warmth, and suitable clothing in the early pages of chapter two.

The general principles of good stretching, at a glance:

In stretches permitting comparison of left and right sides, begin with the tighter side, stretch the looser side, and restretch the tighter side.

When stretching matched pairs of muscles which require the contraction of one of the pairs to produce the stretch in the other, you will benefit from repeating the first side's stretch briefly, to relax the last used muscle group.

When returning from any extended (stretched) position, use muscles other than the ones you have been stretching.

Use the contraction component of the C–R approach to focus the stretch closely on the desired muscles; this occurs through deactivation of the stretch reflex effected by doing work at the end of the normal range of movement.

Always bend forwards after bending backwards.

Always hold the final position of a stretch for five (or sometimes ten) breaths. *If you cannot, you are overdoing the stretch.*

CHAPTER TWO

REHABILITATION STRETCHING EXERCISES

We all know what stretching a muscle feels like. Everyone stretches some part of his or her body every day, even if this is only some mostly instinctive movement done while thinking about something else. What I want to do in this section is try to be more explicit about ways of thinking about stretching, and to discuss an approach which will help you to stretch more effectively.

Limits

Think about stretching for a moment. What does it mean? For most people it means moving some part of the body in a particular direction until it won't move any further. Moreover, this is accompanied by certain sensations—sometimes pleasant, and sometimes not. What stops you stretching beyond a certain point? One constraint is structural: if you are stretching your arm across (in front of) the body at shoulder height for example, no matter how flexible you are you will not be able to stretch past the point where the arm meets the front of your neck. Similarly, once the heel is against the bottom, the knee joint will close no further. However, these structural limitations are not usually the limits you have in mind when you feel you cannot stretch any further.

Another constraint is often called the "stretch reflex." When a muscle is stretched past a certain point, stretch receptors located in particular muscle fibers send signals to surrounding muscle fibers and cause them to contract, with the result that further elongation of the whole muscle stops. It is probably the contraction of the muscle fibers in their maximally lengthened state that causes the sensation you feel when stretching, and that will become pain if you go beyond this point. Some anatomists believe that the main function of this reflex is to protect the associated joint from being overstretched. Specifically, they mean that the ligamentous and bony integrity of any joint has limits constrained by its particular arrangements, and they infer that one of the functions of the stretch reflex is to protect this integrity. These mechanisms help us to avoid serious injury.

Although this protective function may be useful in the normally flexible individual, for most adults this stretch reflex restricts further movement long before the safety of the joint is threatened. The range of available movement decreases with age, and I believe that a stretch reflex being triggered inappropriately early in a joint's range of movement is responsible for much of this loss of flexibility, and much of the muscle tension and accompanying pain experienced in daily life. How might this inappropriate reflex develop?

The answer lies in an extremely complex relationship between the central nervous system and the length and tension of the muscles it governs. Repeated patterns of stimulation form the stretch reflexes. Lifestyle patterns alter as we mature, usually becoming increasingly sedentary. Activities that form these reflexes in their youthful patterns are reduced, and body weight usually increases. These tendencies reinforce each other; and the stretch reflexes reflect these changes. In most people there are no significant physiological constraints to prevent the retention of the flexibility patterns of youth. It is merely that we change our patterns of use as we age and our reflex patterns change to reflect these changes. Physiologically, the most often repeated or strongest patterns of stimuli are remembered best by the body. In sport, this fact forms the basis of most training: that is, repetition leads to enhanced performance. The unfortunate fact of modern life is that the most strongly reinforced patterns of most people's lives do not enhance performance in any way at all.

Another limitation to stretching is the nature of the material being stretched. Tendons and ligaments have very limited extensibility—muscles are the things we stretch. Most muscles can contract to somewhere between 50% and 70% of their normal resting length, and be stretched to about 130%. Stretching beyond this exceeds the elastic limit of the muscle fibers and will cause changes which may not be reversible in the short term. Injury results, and the muscles and associated structures need time to return to normal. This brief account does not consider the differences in forces and effects that muscles experience under fast and slow stretching regimens. The extent to which these differences are pertinent to neck and back pain will be considered below. Before we begin the exercises, let us briefly consider the different methods we may employ to become more flexible. There are two types of stretching: static stretching, which is most commonly recommended, and ballistic (or dynamic) stretching.

Static stretching

In static stretching, a limb is moved into the stretch position and held statically (without movement), usually for a minimum time of somewhere between 10 and 30 seconds. It is often suggested that a number of repetitions of the static stretch be performed. Reasons given to support recommendations for static stretching are that it is safe, and, if done carefully, does not tend to aggravate any existing injuries.

The disadvantages of this conservative approach are that, in the untrained individual, the end point of the stretched position is difficult to determine. By this I mean that it is hard for a beginner to distinguish between the point at which stretching occurs and the further point at which injury may occur. If someone has a problem in a particular area, there is a very natural tendency to hold and protect the area to avoid stretching sensitive tissues. Frequently, moving the body into a position of stretch will elicit the very pain you are trying to remedy.

The "end-point" problem and the tendency towards protecting a sore area have two consequences: either you do not stretch far enough—and hence you will not improve—or you will not acquire an enhanced sensitivity to the region of movement which exists between stretch and injury. I call this the "stretch window." How this window may be opened is dealt with below.

Ballistic stretching

In ballistic stretching, stretching is achieved by momentum, exemplified by kicking as high as possible to the side or the front, as in football or the dance known as the "cancan." The disadvantages of this approach are well known: the risk of injury through momentary over-stretching can be high, depending on the speed and power employed. This sort of movement in sporting activities is the most frequent cause of shoulder and hamstring injuries, because the end point of the movement is so hard to control if significant momentum is employed, and when passions are running high we ignore the warning signs. In any method of stretching, by definition, we are moving part of the body beyond its normal active range of movement. Using momentum to stretch results in less active control for two reasons. One is that the mechanisms that sense position and stretch are less sensitive outside the normal range of movement and, also, are less sensitive at speed. The other is that, once outside the normal range of movement, one's capacity to exert muscular force drops markedly, so that even if you suddenly feel that you are going too far, you may not be able to stop yourself. For these reasons, with exceptions noted below, I do not recommend ballistic stretching as a method for becoming more flexible.

The Posture & Flexibility approach to stretching

This is the name given to my method for improving flexibility and awareness. *Posture & Flexibility* comprises three elements:

(i) a *contract–relax* approach to increase flexibility, within a structure of (ii) *partial poses*, which may be (iii) *partner-based*. I shall address the elements in turn, beginning with a brief history of the "contract–relax" technique, drawn from proprioceptive neuromuscular facilitation (PNF).

(i) *Contract–relax (C–R)*

PNF is a detailed set of patterns for reeducating the neuromuscular responses. PNF was developed at the Kabat-Kaiser Institute during the late 1940s in the United States. What is sometimes called "PNF stretching" today is a tiny fragment of a much larger set of techniques that rely on complex patterns of movement designed to reeducate the movements of people with cerebral or spinal injuries. The description of what is called the contract-relax (C–R) technique, one of three stretching techniques in the original textbook (and what most people mean when they use the term PNF stretching), is but a short paragraph on page 98 (Knott & Voss, 1968). I have taken this C–R fragment from the original PNF system and refined it over the past 15 years, and feel confident that I can offer it now as part of a fully developed method for stretching.

At its most basic, the C–R approach we use means moving the limb into a gently stretched position, and holding it there for a short time (generally 10 to 30 seconds) until you relax and become accustomed to the feeling of being in this position. Then you *contract*—this means that you will push (or pull) the limb back *in the opposite direction to the movement used to get into the stretch position*, for somewhere between six to ten seconds; then you stop pushing. The final part of the approach requires you to restretch the same muscles (as a separate action); the new position is then held, from ten seconds to about a minute. The three parts make up one iteration of the C–R approach. In certain instances, this may be repeated, up to a maximum of three times. We have found that there is no significant improvement with further iterations in any particular stretching session.

One advantage of using the C–R approach to stretching is that it develops strength at the extremes of any range of movement. This is because the contractions increase strength through the isometric principles, covered in chapter three. Thus, not only do you become more flexible, you become stronger as well, especially in the extreme ranges of movements that are left unaltered by conventional approaches to strength or flexibility training.

The original PNF textbook does not specify how much effort to use in the contraction phase. As the techniques were developed for rehabilitation, we may assume that, in general, the therapists were dealing with relatively weak patients. When we are using the C–R technique, how hard should we contract the muscles? Experimenting with willing students and patients over the years has resulted in the following suggestions.

Presuming that you have had neck or back pain, *always* err on the side of not pushing or pulling hard enough when first trying the method, for two reasons. Assuming that we are using the C–R approach to stretch a sore area, the first consideration is that we wish to avoid over-stressing the very muscles we believe to be responsible for the pain. The second is that by being careful and "listening" to the body's responses to a new demand, we are in a position to modify the demand as necessary.

The best way to determine how much effort to use is to push back slowly (over a few seconds) against the resistance until you can actually *feel* the muscle the particular exercise is designed to stretch. Aim to contract with only 20-30% of your maximum effort. In the beginning, we want to open the stretch window to a point between the kind of stretch sensation we judge as desirable, and what we judge is too much and that could be injurious or painful. This requires a deal of sensitivity, and people who have been in pain for a long time have lost much of the ability to make such judgments. However, work slowly and sensitively and you will be working safely. *Err on the side of pushing too little rather than too much.* We are trying to reeducate the body into being more supple—we are not trying to force it into being more supple.

As you become accustomed to working with your body, you may increase the effort expended in the contraction phase. Do this either by contracting more forcefully or by holding the contraction for a longer period. In the case of the hamstring muscles, for example, in time you may find that contractions of 10 to 20 seconds give the best results. With longer contractions, increase the effort *slowly* over five to ten seconds until you reach the desired maximum. Do not contract with more than about half the available effort as we have found this will not increase the stretch effect and the extra effort will leave you feeling more sore the next day. The chance of injuring the back muscles (which have to do increased work to support the stretching position of the trunk as you contract the leg muscles more) also increases beyond this point. However, with the muscles of the neck, which are much smaller and shorter than the muscles of the leg, often only a brief contraction (of a few seconds) will be sufficient to have the desired effect. Work slowly and cautiously, and soon you will find the right contraction force for each muscle group.

To summarize, I do not recommend the ballistic approach as the first choice to increase flexibility because of the inherent danger. Static stretching (exemplified by yoga) is effective. However, it is relatively inefficient in terms of results gained for time spent, has no specific strengthening component at the end of the range of movement, and lacks the capacity to immediately reduce tension in unusually tight muscles.

The C–R approach has a number of important advantages over the static and dynamic approaches. Because you are required to perform an isometric contraction, the muscles involved become stronger at the point in the range where they are usually weak (relative to their strength in the normal range). The action of doing work in the extended position also increases your awareness of the stretching sensation, in effect widening the window between stretching and injuring.

Finally, your flexibility improves markedly as you use the technique; this is due to the stretch reflex being deactivated momentarily due to the activation of *Golgi tendon organs* located at the junction of muscles and tendons whose action is to reduce the contractions in the fibers being stretched, and also perhaps due to the release of "trigger points" in such muscles (Travell & Simons, 1983, vol. 1, p. 89). But this level of detail is unnecessary here—we only need to know that there is a sound set of reasons underlying the approach.

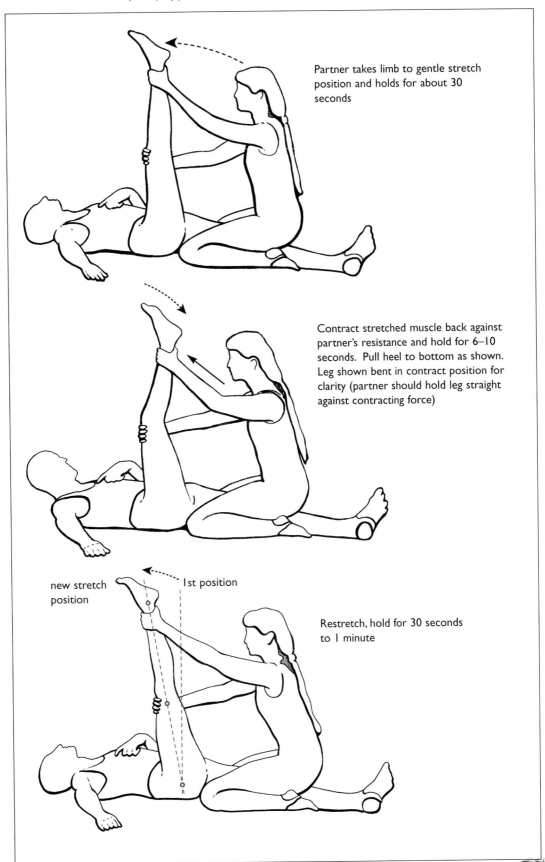

Partner takes limb to gentle stretch position and holds for about 30 seconds

Contract stretched muscle back against partner's resistance and hold for 6–10 seconds. Pull heel to bottom as shown. Leg shown bent in contract position for clarity (partner should hold leg straight against contracting force)

new stretch position

1st position

Restretch, hold for 30 seconds to 1 minute

(ii) *Partial poses*

The second element in my *Posture & Flexibility* approach is that complex movements or whole poses (from yoga, gymnastics, or dance) are broken down into an elemental vocabulary of what I call "functional units of flexibility." I do this to isolate a student's problem areas, and for teaching convenience. These functional units are logical elements, initially based around individual joints, progressing to multiple joints with complex movements as the student improves. Thus, a movement that requires flexibility in a number of areas simultaneously (for example, a forward bend) is broken down into calf muscle stretches, a couple of different hamstring muscle stretches, a hip stretch, a lower back stretch, and so on. Each stretch is done in turn and finally the whole movement is performed for its holistic benefits.

Focusing on specific areas of the body, accompanied by a simplified description of the anatomy involved, helps the student to visualize and feel the parts concerned and how they are integrated into the whole body. Any increase in awareness of these essential aspects aids improvement. Although the goal is to acquire whole-body suppleness, the initial focus is on improving those problem areas located by the partial poses—different for each student. This approach yields the quickest overall improvement. A tight area, even if quite small, profoundly limits more complex positions. Attention to these areas accelerates the acquisition of whole poses. In the class situation, breaking the poses down into smaller parts has the additional advantage that all students can do some of the parts, at least, which improves their confidence greatly.

(iii) *Partner-based*

The third element of the *Posture & Flexibility* approach is partner stretching. The most important advantage of using a partner in your stretching is that you do not need to supply the effort to hold yourself in any particular position. This means that you can relax in the position and attend to your breathing far more easily. Being supported by a partner means that when doing the pushing-back (contraction) part of the exercise, you can concentrate your attention in that particular muscle. The partner can keep a close eye on the *form* of the exercise—*the* crucial aspect.

We must not ignore the psychological aspects either. Doing stretching exercise with another provides support, regularity in practice, and encouragement when needed. Some authors warn of the danger of being stretched by another, but this potential problem has been largely overcome in my system, and will be covered in detail in the exercises below. Choose someone close to your size and weight, and someone with whom you can communicate well. Your partner needs to be sensible and sensitive.

How to breathe

A final point concerns breathing during the stretching process. Contracting the muscles as an aid to stretching is hard work, and naturally your breathing rate will increase during this phase. For this reason, the direction "to take a deep breath in before stretching" is doubly significant, for not only does it signal to the body that you are about to stretch, but breathing deeply will help your breathing and pulse rates to return to normal much more quickly. Changing your breathing patterns during the different phases of the stretching process also helps the body and the mind learn the essential *relaxation* aspect. Electromyograph studies have shown that tension increases slightly in all the muscles in the body each time you breathe in, and reduces slightly each time you breathe out. By focusing your attention on a breath out each time you stretch, you will enhance this natural physiological action. You cannot force muscles to relax and you cannot force them to stretch. You can however *teach* them how to behave more as you wish, and the C–R method combined with focus on breathing is the best I know for this. Accordingly, before you begin the final relaxing, stretching phase of any exercise, you should take a deep breath and make the stretching effort as you breathe out. In time, becoming conscious of breathing in and out provides a focus for more advanced techniques, covered in chapter five.

The final point to make at this stage about breathing is to note that breathing in particular ways can help the *form* of a pose too. For example, breathing in will help you straighten your back, and the directions for some exercises will ask you to "lift the chest." Breathing in at this time makes this direction easier to follow. On other occasions, the directions may ask you to breathe *out* as you get into the position. Usually this will be to empty the lungs momentarily to facilitate bending forward or twisting. Please pay close attention to these suggestions.

Benefits of warmth

The body is more supple when warm. We can use this knowledge to help us stretch. If the body is particularly stiff, have a hot bath before commencing the workout. Research in Germany in the 1960s indicated that the flexibility of any joint was increased 15–20% if the core temperature of the muscles was raised one to two degrees Centigrade. This is easily achieved by soaking in a hot bath. A bath is far more effective than a shower for this purpose because the hot water is in constant, relatively still, contact with the body and this facilitates heat transfer. Afterwards, dress in clothes that permit free movement but retain the heat (for example, cotton tracksuit pants and top).

Why photographs?

The last point I wish to make before we begin is that I have chosen to demonstrate the exercises myself with Jennifer, and with photographs, for two reasons. Most recent books on stretching exercises use line drawings to represent the recommended positions. This is unsatisfactory because a drawing can be made to show any position—hence one does not derive any sense of confidence from a drawing. A photograph conveys the shape and form of a position, but it does a lot more besides. You can see many fine details, such as the position of hands and feet, the precise shape of the back, and so on. There is the reassurance that the exercise really is possible, and that the person writing the book does the exercise too.

Please examine the photographs and the accompanying text carefully before attempting any exercise, *and follow the text and order of the exercises as they are presented.* Important information is included with each of the exercises, so please read the description in full while referring to the accompanying photographs before attempting them. *Do not rely on the photographs alone.*

REHABILITATION

LOWER BACK EXERCISES

1. Seated forward bend

Ensure that you read all directions for the exercise, including how to get out of the final position, before attempting it.

Let us imagine that your back is sore at this very moment. Probably the last thing you want to do is move it at all. Perhaps the usual stretching exercises do not make you feel secure—you feel too vulnerable moving into extended positions, and you feel that you may hurt yourself getting out of the position. If so, this first exercise is for you: it is designed to give a gentle stretch to the entire lower back region.

The exercise is done with the support of your arms at all times, so if you feel you are going too far you can move yourself back to the starting position by arm strength alone, thereby avoiding any additional stress on the lower back. You are in control at all times. You will need a non-sliding chair that is strong enough to support your weight, preferably without arms, and a support on the floor between your feet. This may be a strong box, a couple of large thick books, a footstool or the like.

The **easiest** version is shown in the first photograph. Here, the exercise is performed with a support, two bricks. Use a higher support if you think it necessary; you need to be able to lean forward far enough to be able to place all your weight on the support. Sit on the forward edge of the chair, with your weight evenly placed on both bottom bones, and with your feet placed squarely and securely on the floor slightly in front of the knees. Support the weight of the upper body with the hands on the knees. The back muscles should be completely relaxed, and all weight resting on the arms. Slowly (take a few seconds) let the chin go as far forward in the direction of the chest as is comfortable. This instruction is to initiate a forward bend in the upper back, and to initiate a stretch in the spinal cord. Leaning on the arms, let both arms bend slowly, allowing the body to incline forwards from the waist. (A technical note here. When doing this exercise correctly, both the spine and the hip joints will be involved; this occurs any time the body

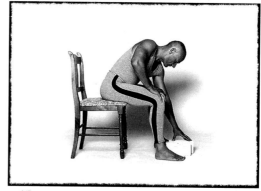

1 Easiest

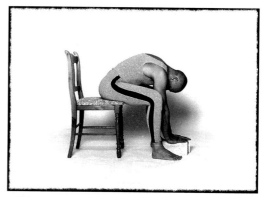

3 Intermediate

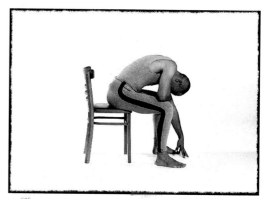

4

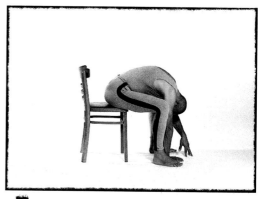

2

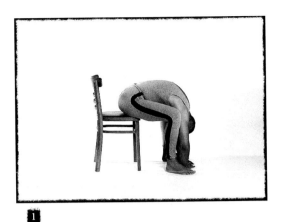

1

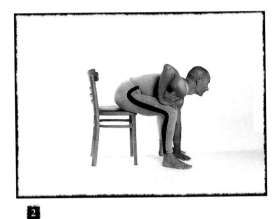

2

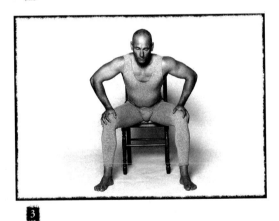

3

Notes

don't hold your breath

lower yourself by your arms

lift yourself up by your arms

you must support yourself
at all times

moves forward between the legs.) At this time, your breathing should be completely normal—do not hold your breath for any reason. Although it may be natural to do so (perhaps in anticipation of pain or because of the newness of the movement) please resist this temptation.

Caution: if at any time you feel that you must return to the beginning position, use your arms to do so. Do not pull yourself back to the starting position with the muscles you are trying to stretch, the back muscles.

When sufficiently forward, take all your weight on one arm without letting the body rotate, and bend the other elbow. Now let the first arm bend and support all your weight on the elbow of the second arm. Bend the first arm now, and place it on the other leg; now you are supporting your weight evenly on both elbows. Rest for a while. Notice that although you are probably already stretching the lower back a little at this stage, because you are taking the weight on your arms, there is little or no pain.

Now we begin the real stretch. If you feel comfortable in this position, support your weight again on one elbow, and reach down to the support with the fingertips of the other arm. Rest this hand on the support. Taking your weight on this hand, bring the other down from your leg and rest on both hands now. Again breathe normally, perhaps with the emphasis on slightly deeper breaths than normal, but at an unhurried, unstressed rate. Take stock of what you feel—you should feel a pleasant stretching feeling in the lower back, but not pain.

Keeping your hands on either the support or the floor, very slowly and gently unweight your arms until you feel a mild stretch in the lower back. You may not need to unweight the arms from the support very much at all in the beginning to achieve a sufficient degree of stretch. Let me stress the point: you must be careful, and move slowly—only you can know how far is enough. Always err on the side of caution. Stay in the final position for a minimum of ten breaths in and out. Do not hurry your breathing. Even though the position may feel awkward, try to breathe normally.

To return to the start position, lift the head up until you are looking forward, rest on one hand, and place the other hand in a support position on your leg. Breathe in, take all your weight on this arm, bring the other into a similar support position, and lift yourself back to the original sitting position with both arms. Now let the breath out, and relax there for a moment.

The **intermediate** version provides a stronger stretch, by having the floor as the support.

This is the first exercise, and may be done whenever the lower back feels tight, even in the office. In addition to the stretch in the lower back, you may also feel a stretch in the muscles at the back of, and inside, the legs, and the bottom muscles. All the muscles on either side of the spine, and from the top of the hips to the lower back, can be stretched using this exercise. Refer to the diagram for details of the muscles involved.

As an aside, anthropologists have noted that indigenous peoples suffer a low incidence of back pain compared with the peoples of the developed world. Of the many different aspects of their lifestyles, one aspect worth noting is that the usual way of holding discussions in these countries is to squat with the heels on the ground, rather than standing around as we do. The squatting action is a good stretch for the muscles stretched in exercise 1 and the ankles (see also exercise 30), and you may care to try it yourself. If your ankles are insufficiently flexible to allow you to balance in the position with your heels on the floor, try holding onto something secure in front of you as you bend the legs. Breathe normally once in the squat position. To increase the stretch in the lower back, you may incline the body forwards from the squat position.

Apart from the effect in the ankles, exercise 1 duplicates many of the effects of squatting (in particular the reversal of the normal lumbar lordosis) and may be done conveniently while at work. I will suggest a list of exercises that may be done in a chair at work in the section entitled "Planning a stretching routine," at the end of this chapter.

For an advanced version of exercise 1, see exercise 22.

Muscles stretched in exercise 1

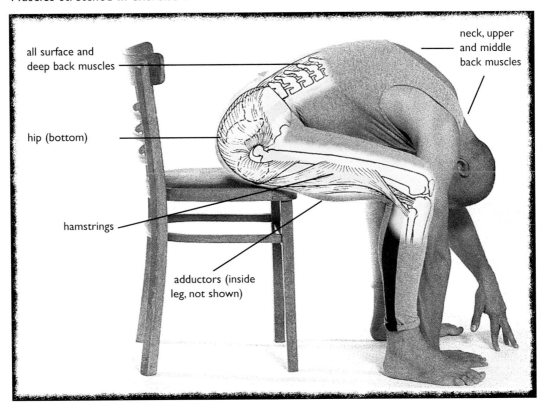

all surface and
deep back muscles

neck, upper
and middle
back muscles

hip (bottom)

hamstrings

adductors (inside
leg, not shown)

2. Seated side bend and rotation

So far, we have stretched mainly the muscles on either side of the spine, the bottom and the back of the legs. The next exercise emphasizes the muscles that run from the top of the hip bones to the spine, and the side muscles of the waist. The final part of the movement, which involves a rotation of the shoulders with respect to the hips, moves this latter stretch from the side of the waist to the muscles closer to the spine itself. The exercise also uses a chair but with one side of the chair placed next to a wall. Make sure that the chair will not slide sideways away from the wall. Place the support close to the ankle next to the wall.

In the **easiest** version, lean forward and reach one hand down to the support, as shown. Keep the head in line with the shoulders. If your back is tender, let yourself down into this position by using the other hand, as for the previous exercise. Lean all your weight onto the support, and roll the other shoulder backwards until it is over the support arm, or as close as you can come to this position. You can press back against the wall to help you get into the first position. Feel the stretch in the side of the waist. Still leaning on the arm, raise the free arm and reach out in the direction of the leg you are leaning over, as shown. You can control the stretch either by the degree of reaching with the top arm, or by how much the lower arm lets the body lean to the side. Doing this will increase the stretch in the side of the waist. Make sure that you are safely supported at all times.

The next time you do the exercise, you can increase all aspects of the stretch by using a lower support. It may be that you feel insufficient stretch in the desired places if supported in the manner described. If so, the hand may be placed directly on the floor—the **intermediate** position; this will give the maximum stretch effect (see photograph on opposite page). All other instructions will be the same. Do not try the more extreme versions if the first version outlined above is effective. As in most exercises, the proportions of one's body determines the strength of the effect.

Assuming that you are in one of the positions outlined, to move the stretch closer into the spine at the same time as maintaining (or even increasing, if this feels safe) the sideways stretch, very slowly roll the top shoulder *forwards* (away from the wall) in small increments. As you do this, you will feel the stretch move from the side of the waist to the muscles closer to the spine. When you have stretched sufficiently (but certainly no less than 30 seconds or so) return the top hand to its starting position (a similar position on the other knee), carefully transfer your weight to your hands, and use the arms to return to the starting position.

Repeat for the other side. Take particular notice of whether one side of the body is more flexible than the other. If this is the case, next time you

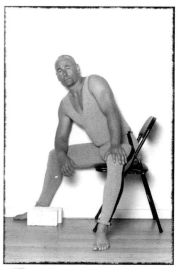

1   easiest

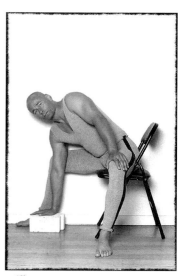

2

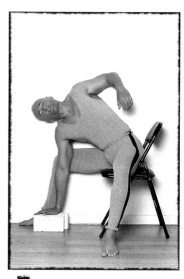

3

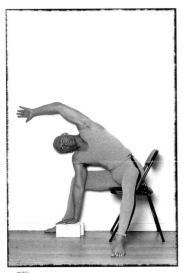

4

stretch begin with the tighter side, then stretch the looser side, and restretch the tighter side. This is a general rule for all exercises that permit comparison of right and left.

For an advanced version of the side-bending component of exercise 2, see exercise 10; for an advanced version of the rotation component, see exercise 24.

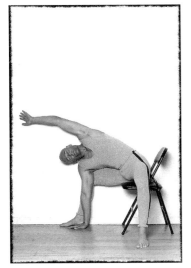

intermediate

Notes

weight evenly on both feet

breathe *in* to roll shoulder back

breathe *out* to stretch arm out

breathe normally in final position

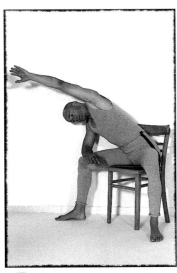

1 alternate support position

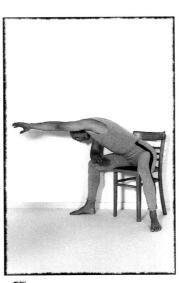

2

3. *Lying rotation*

The third exercise is done on the floor, preferably carpeted or an exercise mat. Stretching on a bed is not suitable because the surface does not usually provide sufficient support. Lie on your back. If lying on your back in this position is painful, try getting into it this way. Lower yourself into the lying position, but keep both knees bent (flexed). Use your arms to hold the knees for additional support. Clasp one knee to the chest (refer to the photographs). When secure, lower the other leg until the back of it is on the floor. Getting into the start position this way avoids arching (or, technically speaking, hyperextending) the lower back. Clasping one knee to the chest maintains a little forward curve in the lumbar spine and this will avoid the pain often associated with lying in a face-up position.

You are now ready to begin the **easiest** version of the exercise. Gently pull one knee towards the chest, and see what that feels like. Some people trap the tendons and muscles of the hip flexors if they pull the knee straight back to the chest, however. If you feel an uncomfortable pinching sensation in the groin of the bent leg, check to see whether overly-tight material around the top of the leg is the cause. If loosening the cloth does not remove the irritation, let the leg go away from the chest until at arm's length, and let it move more to the side of the body. Then bring the knee back to the body again, but this time in the direction of the armpit. Bringing the knee towards the body but more from the side usually avoids the sensation of compression in the hip joint.

Now, gently pull the knee into the chest (or armpit) using both hands as shown. You may feel the stretch variously from behind the leg (top part of the hamstring muscle) to inside the leg (the *adductors*), and you may also feel the stretch in the bottom muscles on the bent-leg side.

After holding the stretch for about ten breaths, let the leg go to arm's length. Hold the outside of the thigh with the hand of the opposite shoulder, as shown. Roll the leg across the body. As soon as it passes over the vertical center-line of the body, take some weight on the bottom leg, and *shift the bottom hip across in the opposite direction*. This ensures that the spine, as seen from above, remains straight. Most floor rotation exercises do not include this refinement, and as a result the spine is both rotated and hyperextended (arched) in the final position, the two movements together often being

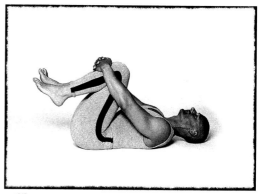

1 If your back is sore

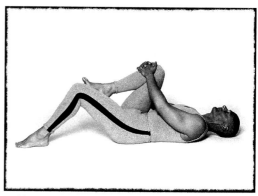

2 Lower one leg at a time

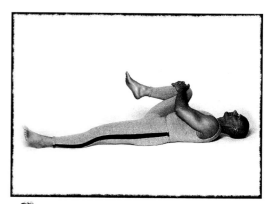

3 Stretch hip

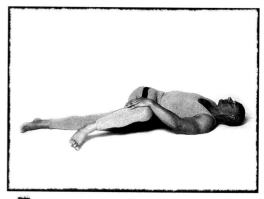

4 Easiest; rest knee on cushion if you wish

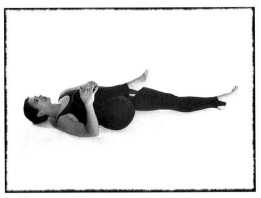

1

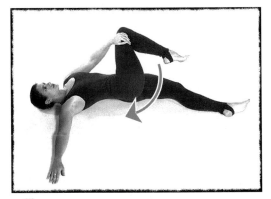

2 Shift bottom hip across and under

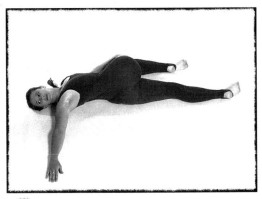

3 Intermediate

Notes

keep shoulders on floor

back straight
(as seen from above)

shift bottom hip under
as you roll across

breathe normally

C–R: press back against hand;
breathe; restretch

sufficient to cause pain in someone with back problems. Generally, it is the extension component of the movement which causes the pain.

Take the top leg across slowly as far as it will go. The limit is when the opposite shoulder begins to lift off the floor. You may hold onto a sturdy table leg to hold the shoulder down, but do not force the stretch. Concentrate on breathing and relaxing. Notice that as you breathe in the leg tends to rise and as you breathe out it tends to go closer to the floor. You may rest the knee of the bent leg on a cushion if the end position is quite a way from the floor (last photo left page). This will enable you to hold the position comfortably.

As you become more flexible, reduce the thickness of the cushion, until it is no longer necessary. Jennifer is demonstrating the **intermediate** version; you will see that her knee is on the ground, and the shoulders are on the floor. Give yourself time, and you will reach this position too. In the exercise, look at your outstretched hand. Hold the final position for about ten breaths, and return the leg to the starting position.

Rather than returning the leg to the floor, bring the other knee up and change your hands over to it, and then let the first leg down to the floor. Again, this will avoid hyperextending the lower back, and make the exercise more comfortable. Repeat all directions for the second leg, taking care to note the tighter side. Next time you stretch, begin with the tighter side, do the looser side, and repeat the movement for the tighter side. In time the two sides will have similar flexibility.

A **Contract-Relax (C–R** for short) version may be tried when you are comfortable with the stretch. In the final stretch position, hold the top leg and very gently try to press it upwards against the resistance of your hand for five seconds or so. Rather than the hip muscles, use the back and waist muscles to press back in order to maximize the stretch in these muscles. Relax, breathe in, and on a breath out, slowly press the leg closer to the floor.

For a more difficult rotation movement, see exercise 24. If you cannot lie on the floor, see exercise 12 for a chair rotation exercise.

4. Partner-assisted lying rotation

At this point I should like to introduce the first partner exercise, which is an assisted version of the exercise you have just done. Do not attempt this partner version before doing the exercise unassisted. Unless you have done the standard version, you will not have a clear idea of your limits, and neither will your partner. If the partner has been watching your effort this far, he or she will be in a good position to assist.

Look at the photograph. You are lying on the floor, in the final position of exercise 3. Your partner is kneeling (on one knee) on the side you are rotating away from. Your partner's other leg is brought up for stability, and the knee placed behind the back of the supporting arm. One hand is holding the shoulder onto the floor, and the other is placed on the top hip, ready to apply a small horizontal force. The partner must be in a stable position, and well balanced. Note the position of the hand on the shoulder: you may have to ask the partner to move the hand more onto the shoulder, or further down the arm until a comfortable position is found. One of the biceps' tendons runs across the front of the shoulder and it may be uncomfortable if much weight is put on it. If this is the case, ask your partner to put a small cushion on your shoulder, and to lean on it. Notice also that the partner has his or her weight more or less directly above the hand holding the shoulder.

You move yourself into the beginning of the stretch position—not the maximum position. Ask your partner to hold you there; that is, the partner's hand placed on the hip does not push the hip further away—it merely rests there as a solid barrier. When your partner is ready, you very gently push the top hip back in the opposite direction (back against your partner's hand) while counting to ten. This is an isometric contraction, or the "contract" part of a "C–R" stretch, discussed previously. Very little effort needs to be used here; it is more of a lean than a push in the early stages. Always be guided by your perception of pain—if it hurts, stop pushing.

Assuming that the pushing part has been completed without a problem, stop pushing. The partner's hand at this stage has remained an immovable barrier against which you have been pushing. The next stage is the taking of a deep breath, after which you **relax** (the "**R**" part) completely, and

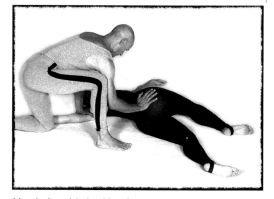

Hand placed *behind* hip for support

Notes

your partner provides
support only

C–R: press hip back
gently to partner's hand

partner must not let you
move during C–R

you must take *yourself* into
new stretch position

relax and breathe normally
in final position

use the arm holding the knee to take the leg a little closer to the floor. The partner, watching and listening to your breathing, leans a small weight horizontally and slowly in the direction indicated, to follow the hip as you take the leg towards the floor. The partner must be very careful at this point, watching your face for any signs of discomfort, stopping if necessary. When a stronger but still comfortable stretch position is reached, the partner holds you there. You remain in the position for the ten-breath count, concentrating on letting any tension go. Imagine the tension is leaving the body with each breath out.

The partner must hold the final position without moving at all. The support provided by the partner must be stable and still, best provided by arranging his or her body so that the effort required can be provided by a leaning force rather than a pushing force. If you feel at all uncertain of the support, you will not permit yourself to relax. It is mainly for this reason that all partner exercises have precise directions to your partner, as well as to you. Repeat all directions for the other side

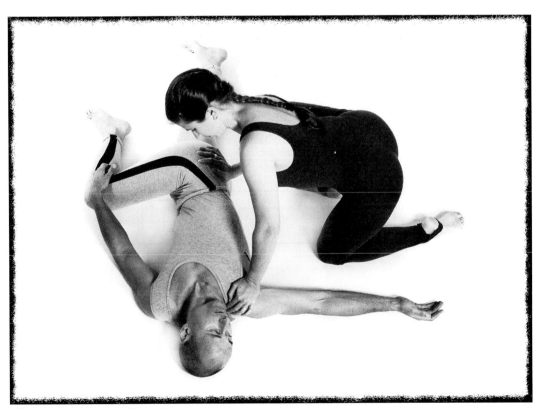

Shoulder held on ground limits final position

5. *Buttock and hip flexor*

Here the focus is the complex of hip and lower back muscles of the front leg mainly, and the hip flexors and part of the thigh muscles of the back leg secondarily. It is an excellent warmup for more difficult exercises, and can give you an insight into left–right differences in flexibility. In the workshops we use it as a simple test for hip flexor tightness—if you find it difficult to straighten the back leg on either side, the hip flexors and the front thigh muscles are likely to be tight.

The **easiest** version (photo 1) uses two bricks as support for the hands. If you needed a block for exercise 1 or 2, use the block for your first attempt in this exercise too. Support yourself on both hands, placed on the inside of the front leg. Place the front foot in front of the knee for stability. Taking the weight of your body on your hands, slowly straighten the back leg (or get it as close to straight as you can). Look to the front (the action of looking forward straightens the upper back). Holding the back as straight as possible, let the arms bend until you feel a stretch in the bottom muscles of the front leg. Let yourself go only as far forward as you can while maintaining a straight back. Do not let the hip of the back leg sink to the floor—the hips need to remain level for best effects. Hold for a few breaths in and out. To this point, you will have confined the stretch to part of the hamstring muscles (long head of *biceps femoris*), the bottom muscle (*gluteus maximus*), and perhaps the adductor muscles if they are tight. See the illustration for details.

In the **intermediate** version, place your hands directly on the floor in the start position. Pull back on your hands a little without letting them slip along the floor; this action will help to straighten the lower back. Let your hips sink to the floor while keeping them level.

The **advanced** part of the movement stretches the muscles of the lower back as well. Take a breath in, check that the hips are level, and as you breathe out, let the arms bend further and also let the head go forward until the lower back is stretched too. Hold the final position for a few breaths in and out. This position is strenuous, and the supporting arms will be working hard. To come out of the position, always take a breath in and hold it in until you stand up. This will reduce the tendency to feel

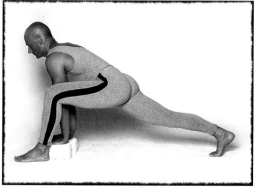

1 Easiest

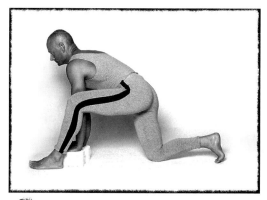

2 Rest on toes of back foot

Notes

use sturdy support

lower hips as far as you can

keep back as straight as you can

try to straighten back leg slowly

keep neck and head neutral

don't hold your breath!

Notes (opposite)

hips level

lower both hips as far as you can

C–R: press front foot into floor

breathe in; relax, breathe out, let arms bend, take body towards floor

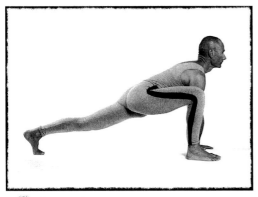

1   Intermediate

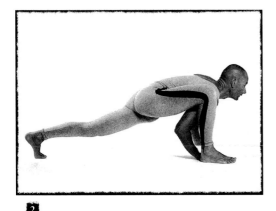

2

lightheaded—always a possibility when doing a difficult movement with the head lower than the heart. Rest for a moment or two before stretching the other side.

The reason the hamstring muscles are not emphasized in this movement (except as described) is because the knee is flexed. Assuming that you can maintain good form to this point, you can increase the stretch in the hamstring muscles in a second stretch by relaxing, moving the front foot further forward (with respect to the knee), and restretching. Do not be tempted to exaggerate the forward placement of the foot.

A **C–R stretch** can improve hip flexibility. In the final stretch position, try to press the front foot into the floor gently. This action engages the illustrated muscles. Hold the contraction for a few seconds and restretch, while holding the hips level to avoid the tendency for the hip of the straight leg to sink to the floor.

Right hip in the intermediate position showing stretched muscles in exercise 5

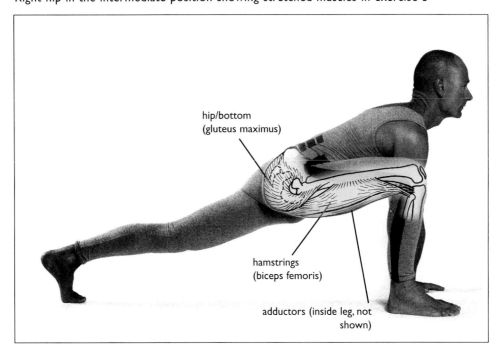

hip/bottom
(gluteus maximus)

hamstrings
(biceps femoris)

adductors (inside leg, not
shown)

6. Seated hip

Inflexible hip muscles (in particular *gluteus maximus*, the main muscles of the bottom, and *piriformis*, one of the external hip rotators) can contribute significantly to back pain in some people, and to dysfunction in many more. This stretch is one of the best to loosen this area. It is offered in three forms. Exercises 6, 7 and 8 all affect the same general area and are effective *piriformis* stretches. Anatomical details are shown in the illustration accompanying exercise 7, page 54.

The **easiest** of the three, and the one which you should use if you are not sure how loose the hip joint is in this movement, begins by sitting on a chair as shown. Ensure that your weight is placed evenly on both bottom bones (the *ischial tuberosities*). This position also relieves any stretch on the sciatic nerve and the hamstring muscles. Wrap the opposite arm around the knee, and take a breath in and sit up straight. Draw the knee as close to the body as you can. The stretch will be felt in the hip of the held leg.

If one hip is tighter in this movement (likely to be the case if you have a leg-length difference) a **C–R stretch** may be used on the tight hip to minimize the difference in function. Gently press the leg away from the body while holding it in the stretched position for a few seconds, and relax completely. Check the back for straightness, and while breathing out, gently restretch the hip by bringing the knee closer towards the body. Hold the final position for five breaths or so. Do not press the knee away from the body with any great force—a gentle press will do the same job with less discomfort.

In the second, **intermediate** version, sit on the floor as shown with one leg outstretched. Bend the other leg at the knee and place the foot on the outside of the straight leg. Check that your back is held straight (lift the chest to make sure), and grasp the knee with the opposite shoulder's arm. As you breathe out, gently bring the knee back to the chest. You will feel the stretch in the hip of the held leg. A C–R stretch can be used here, too. Stretch the other side.

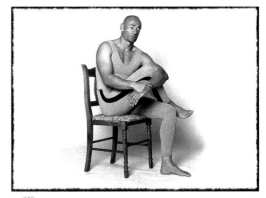

2

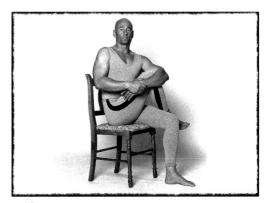

1 Easiest

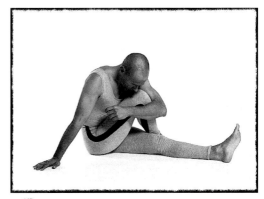

1 Intermediate

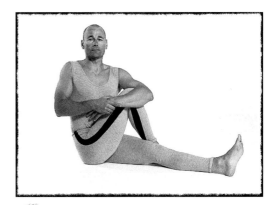

2

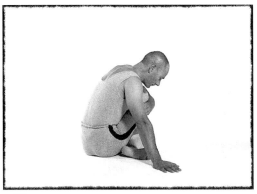

1 Advanced

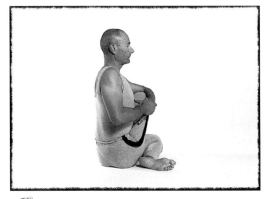

2

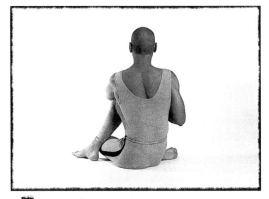

3 Lower back straight

In all respects other than the starting position, the **advanced** version is the same as the second. Look at the photograph. Do not sit on the folded lower leg, but keep it sufficiently outside the line of the body to permit both bottom bones to contact the floor firmly. Because this is an important point, you may wish to try this version sitting on a hard floor without any mat or cushion the first few times you try the exercise. Move subtly from side to side in the starting position until you are sure that both bones are pressing on the floor equally. Follow the directions for the above exercise, including those for the C–R component.

Notes

lift chest to straighten back

keep *both* buttocks
on the support

draw knee to side of chest

C–R: press knee against
inside of forearm

breathe normally in final position

7. Lying hip

Due to the course of the *piriformis* muscle through the pelvis and the normal differences in attachment points in the general population, the one exercise cannot be guaranteed to have the same effect on everyone. Accordingly, you will need to try all the *piriformis* exercises to find the right one (or two) for you. Even a slightly different joint position in an exercise can yield a very different stretch sensation, even though the same muscle is involved. For this reason, if you suspect that *piriformis* is involved in your problem, make sure you try all related exercises: exercises 6, 7, and 8. Exercise 26 is an advanced version.

Lie on the floor face-up as shown, with your legs bent. Place the ankle of one leg on the thigh of the other, near the knee. If your lower-leg bones are relatively short, place the outside of the foot on the thigh rather than the ankle, for we want the knee of this leg to be out to the side as far as practical. Reach *through* your legs and hold the front of the knee of the first leg, or (depending on the length of your arms in relation to the length of your torso) slide your fingers in and hold the back of the first leg's thigh instead. Pull the knee back towards the chest until you feel a stretch in the other leg's hip.

A **C–R** version can be effected by pressing the ankle of the leg closest to you into the thigh of the leg you are holding. Press for five seconds or so, stop pressing, and breathe in. Breathe out, relax completely (except for the arms holding the leg), and slowly pull the knee further into the chest. Hold the final position for ten breaths in and out. This will provide a very strong stretch for these muscles. The contraction may be repeated if required, but we have found that doing any more than three C–R stretches in one session does not yield any additional stretch benefits. Once or twice in the beginning is sufficient.

While it is usually the case that muscular problems are experienced in the tighter of a pair of muscles, we have found that this pattern is not as reliable in sufferers of *piriformis* syndrome, especially if found together with leg-length inequality. The significance of this is simply that, even though the hip muscles in the affected leg may be looser than the other in these exercises, relief will be experienced by stretching the muscle further in its range of movement, even if it already demonstrates a greater range of movement than its fellow.

Three ways the sciatic nerve may exit the pelvis

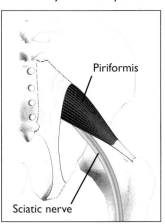

Sciatic nerve passes underneath *piriformis* (most common)

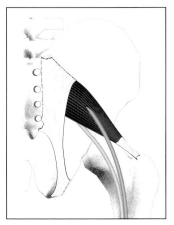

Peroneal or other part of sciatic nerve passes through *piriformis* (20-35% of population)

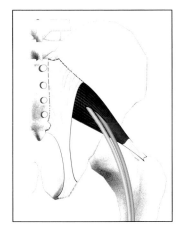

Whole sciatic nerve passes through *piriformis* (rare)

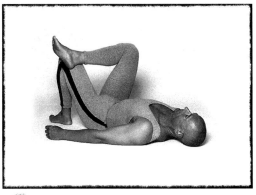

1

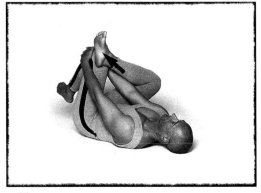

2 C—R direction

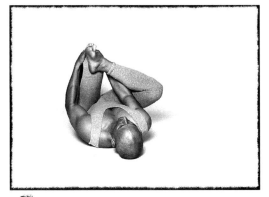

3 Pulling this leg stretches the other

Notes

keep whole back flat on floor

hold *back* of thigh if you can't
hold front of knee

C–R: press closest foot into knee

after breath out, restretch
by pulling leg closer

8. *Table-top hip*

We have found that this version of the *piriformis* stretch may be done quite easily in the work place; in fact anywhere there is a sufficiently strong flat surface, like a table top or bench. Any height is suitable; I am showing it on a low table. Make sure that the surface you use can support your weight on one of its edges safely. I have shown the exercise on a bare table top for clarity.

Place *one* hip on the edge of the table, as shown, with the ankle of the leg on something soft, like a folded towel or a blanket. The reason for this is that if the outside ankle bone presses onto the table without padding, it will be so uncomfortable that you will not be able to concentrate on the stretch in the hip. These details may seem unimportant as you read, but I cannot overemphasize the importance of being comfortable while you work. Anything that distracts you will work against the effectiveness of the final position. Hold the edge of the support with one or both hands, and lift your chest to straighten your back. Let the leg on the table fall to the outside as much as it can; if it is a long way off the surface, though, don't worry—the stretch will still be effective. Holding the back straight, lean forwards *from the hip*. The reason for emphasis is that most people will lean by letting the lower back bend; if you are not sure, ask a friend to check, or set a mirror next to you in a suitable position. Lean until you feel a stretch in a similar place to the previous exercises. Pause there for a moment. If you do not feel the stretch in the desired place, make sure that you are aiming the center of your body to the *sole* of your foot and not to your shin.

The **C–R** stretch is done by using the hip where you feel the stretch to push the ankle *through* the surface of the support. Press down for five seconds or so, making sure that your body does not move at all as you do so. Stop pressing (don't let the body move though), and breathe in. Relax, and restretch by leaning further forwards. When you have sufficient stretch in the hip region, hold the final position for at least 30 seconds (ten breaths at normal speed is around this length of time). Repeat for the other side.

Exercise 26 describes an advanced version of this stretch.

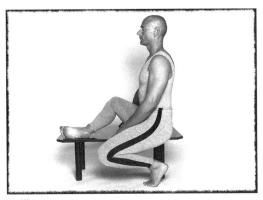

1 To stretch the *right* hip

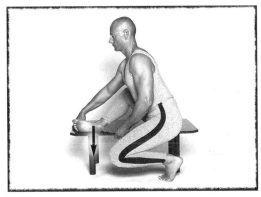

2 C–R direction

Notes

lift chest to straighten back

lean forwards from *hips only*

C–R: press foot into support

breathe, relax, and lean
further forwards

keep back straight

9. Hip flexors

These stretches are very effective for relieving low-back pain, even though they do not stretch the lower back in any way. Exercise 9 stretches a group of powerful muscles, the hip flexors (particularly *psoas major* and *iliacu*s), shown on page 62. These muscles can play a major role in shaping the lumbar curve, especially if the abdominal muscles are weak. Inflexible hip flexors are often the reason why people with back problems cannot lie face-up with legs outstretched without feeling discomfort. These muscle groups are also often implicated in athletes with low-back pain, especially those who use incorrect strengthening exercises for the abdominal muscles (see chapter three). I have shown the partner version first, for having taught these exercises to many thousands of people, I can say that one's natural skill in cheating (or, putting it another way, the very natural tendency to avoid stretching a tight part) means that this is one of the most difficult exercises to learn. The majority of exercises that claim to stretch the hip flexors in fact avoid that very group of muscles, either extending the spine, or stretching some of the thigh muscles. Accordingly, I urge you strongly to learn this exercise with a partner—and learn precisely *where* the stretch should be felt before attempting the solo version shown later in this section.

Anatomically, the action of the hip flexors is to pull the knee to the chest (ignoring the role of the abdominal muscles for a moment). So, to stretch the flexors the thigh needs to be taken backwards with respect to the trunk. Look at the photograph of the starting position: to be specific, the starting position requires that the hip joints be square (at 90 degrees) to the line of the legs or, if sufficiently flexible, the back leg's hip slightly ahead of the other hip, as might be seen from above. The front foot is well in front of the knee, the back leg back as far as you can, resting your weight on the knee. Your hand is placed on your knee for support. The standard variations in how far back the leg can go are illustrated in the top two photos on the facing page. It is desirable to have the back leg's knee on a padded surface to avoid any discomfort to the kneecap. Ask your partner to take a hook grip on the hip bone of the front leg, and to press on the hip of the back leg, behind or below the hip joint on the bottom itself, as shown. This hooking and pressing force induces a rotation into your hips which will

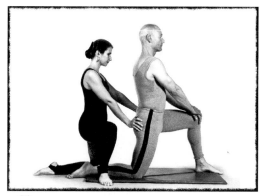

1 Hold with straight arms

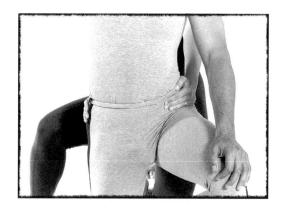

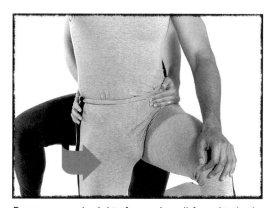

Partner: press back hip forwards; pull front hip back

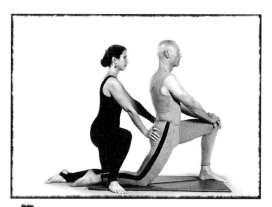

2 Support hand on or *below* hip joint

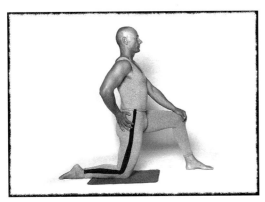

Easiest leg position

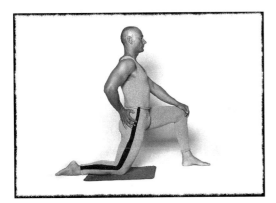

Intermediate leg position

Notes

keep trunk *upright* (vertical)

rotate back hip
forwards all the way

keep shoulders square
to line of legs

press hand on knee
to *tighten* abdominals

C–R: try to drag the
back leg forwards

after breath out, restretch
and hold

counter the tendency for you to lose the stretch in the place you want it. With your hips held in position (with the back hip at least level with the other, and ideally forward, as might be seen from above), let both hips move forward and down until you feel a stretch at the top of the leg, towards the groin. Retention of the alignment is critical to the success of the pose, and your partner will have to work hard to hold the position. Maintain this stretch for a few breaths in and out, and relax into it.

Check your form. If the lower back hyperextends strongly, resulting in an obvious curve backwards, you will need to provide an additional counteracting force. This is done by pressing down firmly on the front knee with your support hand, which will tighten the abdominal muscles. This tilts the top of the pelvis backwards and flattens the arch in the back. As you do this, you will immediately feel an increase in the stretch in the front of the back leg. For the same reason, you must not lean forwards over the front leg. This avoids the stretch by letting the pelvis tilt forwards. Another way to achieve the correct position is to tell yourself to "tuck your tail under" (by tightening the bottom muscles) while in the stretch position. Both suggestions flatten the lumbar curve. If you still find that the stretch tends to increase the lumbar curve rather than stretch the hip flexors, it may be that your partner's hand is too high on the hip, or the abdominal muscle bracing is being lost. This may be because you are not maintaining enough tension in these muscles or because your partner is trying to move you into a stretch position that is too advanced for your present flexibility and abdominal strength. Come out of the stretch, retighten the abdominal muscles, and go into the stretch only as far as you can maintain the correct trunk shape.

The **C–R stretch** is achieved once in the full stretch position by you trying to bring the back leg forwards gently. Your partner will have to increase the pressing effort on the back hip slightly to counter the additional rotational force produced by your efforts: *no movement of your body should occur while contracting*. Hold the contraction for six to ten seconds. Relax, take in a deep breath and, as you breathe out, let the hips (still maintained in the correct position) go a little further forwards and down. Hold the final stretched position for ten breaths. The use of the contraction component focuses the stretch even more closely on the hip flexors, through deactivation of the stretch reflex by doing work at the end of the normal range of movement. Repeat for the other leg, critically comparing right with left.

If one side is tighter than the other, begin with the tight side in your next stretching session, then stretch the looser side, and restretch the tight side once again. In time, you will be able to bring the function of both sides nearer a balance. For some people, the muscles you are trying to stretch become apparent only when you try to bring the back leg forwards in the stretch.

The solo version of the exercise is effective once you know where the stretch should be felt. Look at the photographs. Support yourself by leaning against a smooth wall, so you can slide along it as you go further into the stretch. It is possible to do the stretch without support, but if you are concentrating on balancing the pose will not be as effective. With the back leg's hip rotated forwards (and held in this position for the duration of the exercise), keep the body vertical by placing your one hand on the knee of the front leg, as shown. Place the other hand on the bottom, directly behind the hip joint and with the elbow pointing backwards. Use this hand to push the hip of the back leg forwards as far as it will go—this requires that this hip rotates away from, and in front of, the pushing hand. Let both hips sink in the direction of the floor, only as far as you can maintain both the forward rotation of the back hip *and* the trunk's alignment with respect to the floor. Neither of these constraints may be sacrificed to achieve a lower position.

Sinking towards the floor takes the back leg away behind the body, with the main stretch being felt at the front of the back leg, high up near the hip joint. You may also feel a stretch at the back of the front leg. Remain in the stretch position for the usual ten-breath period, and use the arm on the front leg to help you return to the starting position. Repeat directions for the other leg. A **C–R stretch** may be done in this version, too, by bracing yourself in the final position and trying to drag the back leg forwards. Hold the contraction for six to ten seconds, stop, and take a deep breath in. Check your bracing (are the stomach muscles working and is the back hip forward?) and on a breath out go further forwards. Compare left with right, and the next time you stretch begin with the tighter hip, and stretch it a second time after stretching the other.

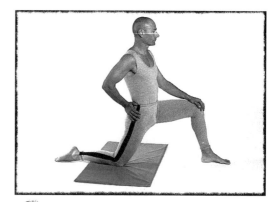

1

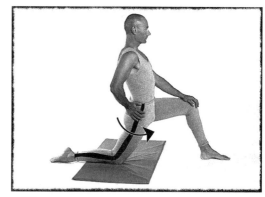

2 Push back leg's hip forwards

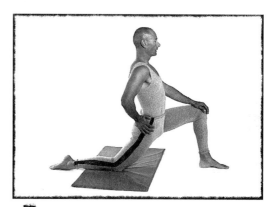

3

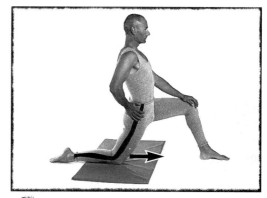

4 *Try* to drag back leg forwards

Notes

lean against wall for support

hold trunk vertical

rotate back hip
forwards all the way

shoulders square
to line of legs

press hand on knee
to *tighten* abdominals

C–R: try to drag the
back leg forwards

breathe in; breathe out; restretch
and hold

I must emphasize that the positioning of the hips with respect to the line of the legs is critical. The most common fault in the performance of this movement is that as the hips move forwards and down towards the floor, the hip of the back leg lags behind (due to tightness in the very muscles we want to stretch) and, in relative terms, it rotates in the opposite direction to the main movement. As this happens, the stretch is moved from iliopsoas to the *quadriceps* or the *adductor* groups (front and inside thigh muscles), thereby rendering the stretch ineffective. Another common fault is that the person lets their trunk incline forwards from vertical as they go into the stretch; this loses the stretch because the pelvis tips forwards in the process, bringing the attachment points of the hip flexors closer to the leg.

Psoas, iliacus (iliopsoas), and quadratus lumborum

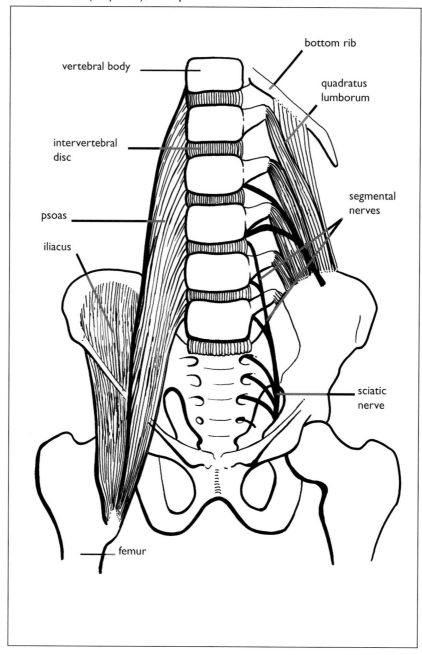

Exaggerated lumbar curve caused by tight iliopsoas

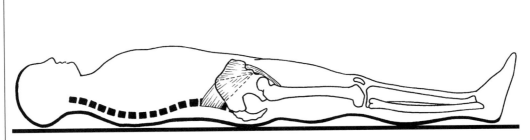

normal length iliopsoas, normal lumbar curve

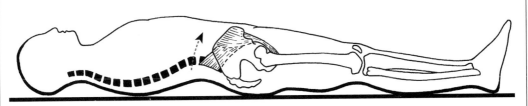

short iliopsoas: spine pulled forward (hyperextended) as legs are lowered, which can make lying face-up uncomfortable. A pillow under the knees flexes hip, and relaxes back.

10. Trunk side bending

In the workshops we have been running nationally in Australia working with thousands of people, we have found that most people's back pain is experienced in a pair of deep lumbar muscles located right next to the spine, named *quadratus lumborum*. Stretching these muscles usually offers immediate relief from the pain. Further, if you have established that you have an effective leg-length difference, it is likely that your back pain is greater on one side, usually the short-leg side. Stretching *away* from this sore area generally gives relief. These muscles are difficult to stretch ordinarily, but if you follow the directions of the next two exercises, you will be able to locate these muscles precisely. The second version (sitting on the floor) is the single most important lower-back exercise for most people.

The **easiest** chair version requires a review of all directions for exercise 2. Do the exercise as directed as a warmup. Look at the first photograph: it shows a more advanced final position of exercise 2. Sit astride a chair in such a way as to allow you to hold the front edge securely, as shown, with the knees spread well apart for stability. Lean *directly* to the side slowly, as far as you can (don't lean forwards or backwards, and don't rotate the shoulders), and hold on to the front of the chair while *hanging* off this arm. Straighten your top arm, and reach out to the side as far as you can; this will increase the stretch considerably. If the shoulder alignment is as described, you will feel a stretch in the side waist muscles (the *oblique* group), and perhaps a small stretch nearer to the spine. To move the stretch closer in to the place you want it, while leaning to the side very slowly *roll* the top arm and shoulder forwards in small increments until you feel the stretch in your sore place. You will find that to maintain the stretch intensity you will need to increase the sideways component slightly. Hold your final position for a few breaths in and out. To return to the starting position, roll the top shoulder further forwards until the stretch disappears, and sit up. Repeat for the other side, and take note of any right/left differences.

The **easiest** floor version is demonstrated first; see photograph 2. To get into the starting position, sit with your back against a wall, with a strap and a rolled-up towel within reach. Move one leg as far as you can sideways towards the wall, without disturbing the position of the hips. Fold the other leg, bringing the foot near the groin.

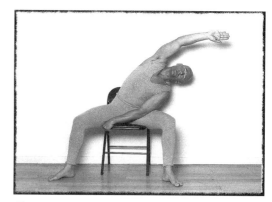

Chair version

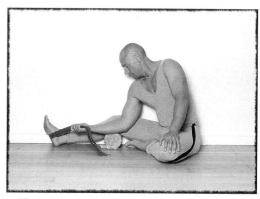

1 Easiest floor version

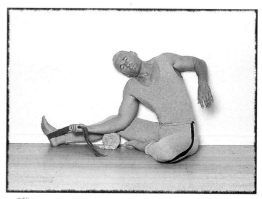

2

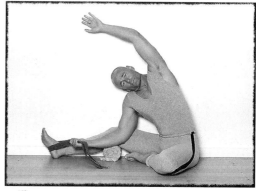

3

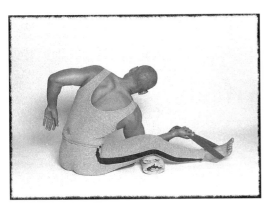

Photo 2, from behind

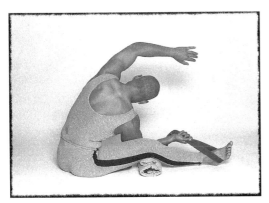

Photo 3, from behind

Notes

lean back against wall

elbow *inside* leg, palm-up

roll top shoulder back

reach top arm out as far
as you can

breathe normally

roll top shoulder *forwards*
to come out of stretch

In this position, move the whole body as little as you need to bring the straight leg against the wall. Getting into position this way is to keep the main movement the body will have to make to get into the next position a *sideways* bend; if you simply sit against the wall with one leg folded (so the hips are at right angles to the wall) the main component of movement towards the leg will be a forward bend, which will be nowhere as effective.

Place the towel under the knee; the tighter your hamstrings , the thicker roll you will need. Loop the strap around the foot as shown. Hold the strap at a length that will permit you to place your elbow on, or near, the floor, *in front of* the leg after leaning to the side. Press this elbow against the inside of the leg, and use the shoulder muscles to press the elbow against the leg to bring this shoulder forwards. Lock yourself into this position. Take a breath in, and on a breath out, slowly *roll* the top shoulder back towards the wall, as far as you can. This movement will stretch the muscles between the hip and the ribs, on the bent-leg side. This may be a sufficient stretch; if not, reach the top arm out in line with the wall as far as you can. Try to breathe normally—one lung is stretched open, and the other is compressed, so breathing will be more difficult than usual. Hold the position for ten breaths. Take a short break, and repeat all directions for the other side. You may feel the stretch in the side of the waist, above the hip, and along the back (and perhaps even inside) the leg you are stretching over.

If you are careful, a **C–R** stretch may be done in this final position. Check your alignment, and grasping the strap firmly, gently pull back on the strap, using the muscles *above the hip* you are stretching away from, for five to ten seconds. Stop, and after taking a breath in, relax your body completely (except for the hand holding the strap), and on a breath out, gently pull on the strap to bring the body a little closer to the leg. Hold the final position for ten breaths or so, and repeat directions for the other side.

The **partner C–R version** is an **advanced** exercise (shown on page 66); accordingly, caution is essential. Although an advanced technique, this version is suitable for beginners if you have a considerate partner, and doing the movements will loosen these muscles in a way which is hard to achieve on your own. The C–R version has two parts—selection of the appropriate part depends on your particular pattern of flexibility.

Not being able to put the shoulders in the illustrated vertical position suggests a restriction in rotation, so have your partner support the bottom shoulder as shown. Notice that the partner's knee is supporting the bottom hand—a partner's position must always be strong and stable. Once in position, try to bring the top shoulder back. When you have reached your limit, your partner holds the top shoulder as shown while supporting the bottom one with his or her other hand. Your partner gently helps to bring the top shoulder back until it is vertical or until the stretch is sufficient; whichever occurs first. Once in the final position, the **C–R stretch** requires you to ask the partner to hold you in position while you try to bring the top shoulder forward a little against this resistance. Hold the contraction for five to ten seconds. Relax completely, and as a separate movement (using a breath out), ask the partner to take the top shoulder back very gently until the desired stretch is felt. Repeat for the other side.

If the vertical shoulders position is not difficult, but the bend over the leg is, then use your partner's assistance in the following way. Look at photograph 4. Here, my partner has placed herself so that she can lend some weight in the direction of the leg I am trying to bend over. This is crucial. In this **C–R version**, position yourself as far in the stretch direction as you can, and when you require the assistance, ask the partner to place his or her hands on the side of your body below the top shoulder, and in line with the leg you are trying to bend over. Once supported, very gently push back against your partner, so that you have to use the muscles of the side of the waist and above the hip. Only push back with a small effort, which you hold for five to ten seconds. Upon relaxing, take a deep breath in, and as you breathe out, ask the partner to lean a fraction more weight on you in the direction of the leg, until you feel the right intensity of stretch. Hold the final position for the usual ten breaths. Repeat for the other side.

Both these exercises stretch the muscles at the side of the waist initially (the *oblique* group), but in time as these muscles loosen, the exercises become a powerful stretch for *quadratus lumborum*. This muscle runs from the top of the hip bone to the sides of all the lumbar vertebrae, and a thin

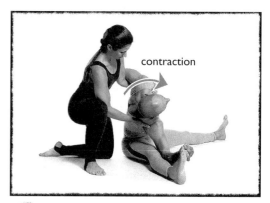
1 C-R to improve rotation

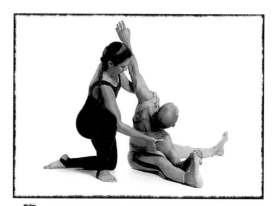
contraction

2

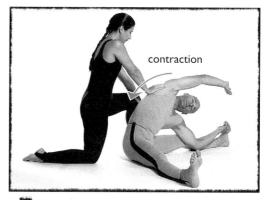
3 C-R to improve side bending

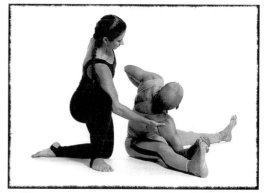
contraction

4

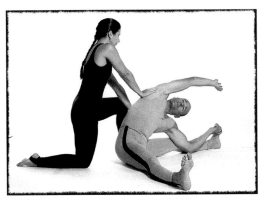

5 Final position

Notes

partner supports bottom shoulder

first C–R: try to pull
top shoulder *forwards*

second C–R: press body directly
away from straight leg

breathe and restretch
in between C–Rs

hold final position for at least
30 seconds

sheet of the muscle runs from the hip bone to the last rib. See the illustration for details. As you stretch further, the muscle groups which run parallel with, and on either side of, the spine (*erector spinae*, not shown) will also be stretched. When the arm is extended, *latissimus dorsi* (the wide back muscles under the arms) is stretched as well. In a very small percentage of people, pain seems to be experienced in the sheet of fascia to which *latissimus dorsi* attaches, and which spans the *sacro-iliac joint*s. If doing the above exercises gets close to your problem area, but the effect is still a little too high, ask a partner to hold the wrist of your extended arm in the final position described above. A **C–R stretch** for *latissimus dorsi* and its *aponeurosis* may be effected by asking your partner to gently pull the arm further out over the leg. Once in the stretch position, gently pull your arm *directly* back to your body for the usual length of time. On a breath out, your partner draws the arm further off the body. To move the stretch further in towards the spine, very slowly roll the top shoulder forwards while your partner maintains the stretch. Once you have found the right angle, do the C–R stretch once more. This stretch can be very effective for apparent *sacro-iliac* pain.

For an advanced standard alternative to these exercises, see exercise 23.

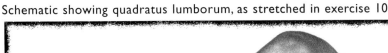

Schematic showing quadratus lumborum, as stretched in exercise 10

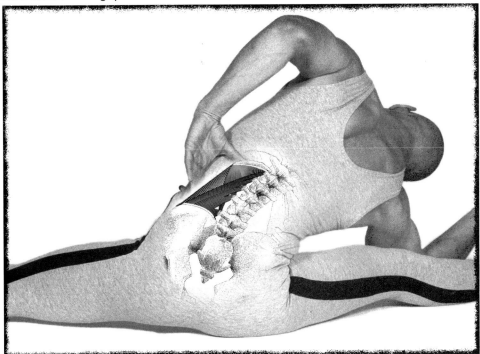

11. Hamstrings

These exercises allow you to concentrate your attention on the hamstring muscles of one leg at a time. The advantage is that the entire strength of the trunk muscles can be used to maintain the straightness of the lower back, and the whole upper body can thus be used as a lever for stretching the hamstrings . The three muscles of the hamstrings hamstrings originate at the *ischial tuberosities* (the two bones we sit on) and run down the back of the thigh and cross the knee joint to finish at the lower leg. For this reason, the leg needs to be straight to stretch these muscles completely. See the illustration for details.

The **easiest** way to learn how to isolate the hamstrings is to begin with the lying partner version. This version of the exercise is recommended even if your hamstring muscles are particularly tight, because the positioning of the body ensures that there is no lower back involvement, and it is easy to hold the final position. The stretch may be felt anywhere between the bottom and the calf muscles on the stretched leg. Lie face-up as shown. Have your partner sit on one of your outstretched legs (but not on the kneecap) and lift the other until you feel a gentle stretch along its length. If your hamstrings are very tight, your leg may only come a little way off the floor (indicated by the shaded outline in the first photograph). The partner must be in a position that permits relaxed and secure support of the lifted leg. Hold this position for half a minute or so.

For a **C–R stretch,** there are two contractions that may be used, affecting different parts of the hamstring group. For the first, use the muscles at the back of the leg to try to flex the leg at the knee (that is, try to pull the heel back to the bottom) for ten seconds or so. Photograph 2 shows the leg bending slightly; this is to illustrate the direction of the contraction—your partner needs to resist this bending movement (Jennifer is applying a hand above my knee for this). Stop pressing, and after taking a breath in, relax the leg completely, and let you partner take the leg a little further in the stretch direction. Hold this new position for 30 seconds. This contraction engages the bulk of the hamstring group.

The second **C–R stretch** requires you to press the leg being held directly down to the floor while keeping the leg straight, for six to ten seconds. Pushing the leg down to the

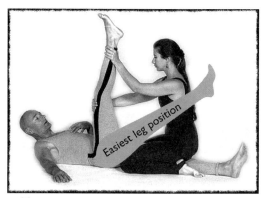

1 Hold leg straight against first C–R

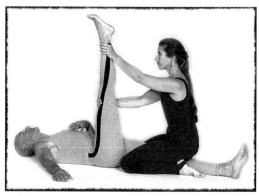

2 Hold leg straight against second C–R

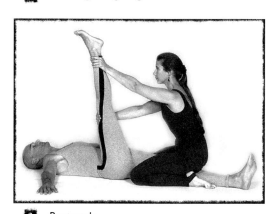

3 Restretch

Hamstring muscle from side; biceps femoris

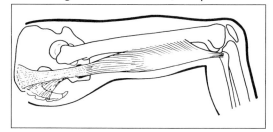

The three hamstring muscles

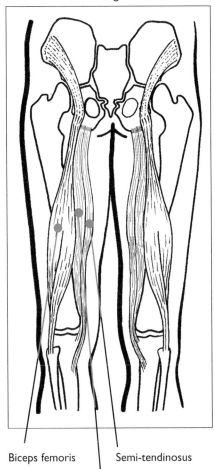

Biceps femoris   Semi-tendinosus

Semi-membranosus

Notes

start position depends
on your flexibility

both buttocks must
stay on the floor

keep your body relaxed

two C–Rs: try to bend knee;
press leg to floor

restretch after breath in and out

floor in this fashion will engage *biceps femoris* mainly. Do not press too hard the first time you try the movement—a third of your strength is about right. Stop pressing, relax completely and take a deep breath. As you breathe out ask your partner to lift the leg very slowly higher until you feel the required stretch. The leg should remain straight (do not let it bend to avoid the stretch), so your partner will need to apply a straightening effort above the knee as shown—this is preferable to you expending energy to hold the leg straight yourself. Relax completely in the stretched position, letting your partner do all the work of holding the leg. Imagine the muscles in which you feel the stretch lengthening and relaxing as you breathe out. Hold the final position for at least ten breaths, and repeat for the other leg. The two contraction, relaxation, and restretch sequences may be repeated for further effect. Always hold the final position for a minimum of ten breaths. ***If you cannot, you are overdoing the stretch.***

The action of stretching the leg further away from the floor also stretches the sciatic nerve, which is often involved in back pain. The sciatic nerve is the longest nerve in the body, and its significance was discussed in an earlier chapter. There is one additional refinement to this exercise. Look at the position of the foot in relation to the leg in your final stretch position. A strongly pointed foot suggests a shortening of the calf muscles. If this applies to you, the stretch can be intensified by asking your partner to apply weight to the ball of the foot to increase the flexion at the ankle in the final stretch position. This action can use a **C–R stretch** effectively. Press the ball of the foot back against your partner's resistance, and restretch. Always do these stretches separately before doing them in sequence. A strongly flexed ankle in the final position of the hamstring stretch is also a maximum stretch for the sciatic nerve. If you suspect that your calf muscles need further stretching, **see exercise 30 for an advanced stretch.**

The **easiest solo version** is illustrated. Sit as shown. Loop a towel or something similar around the foot and hold with both hands. Allow the back to bend a little to find the starting position. Hold the strap tightly, and slowly arch the whole back backwards—it is the straightening action which stretches the hamstrings , by tilting the top of the pelvis forwards. The straightening effort also helps to strengthen the back muscles (by isometric contraction). You may need to ask your partner if your back is straight, as it is a difficult thing for most beginners to feel.

The next most effective form of the exercise is to perform a **C–R stretch** yourself, without support. This can be useful if you are stretching solo. This technique is most effective in preparing for holding a long static stretch. Assuming you are in the final stretch position (photograph 2), check to see if your back is straight—there should be a straight line from the neck to the base of the spine. Pull back gently on the hands as though you are trying to pull the hands and body away from the feet while trying to lift the chest up (this last direction will ensure that your back stays straight). If your form is correct, the only place you will feel any effort is in the hamstring muscles, apart from the straightening effort in the middle back. If you don't feel the effort in the hamstrings , check the straightness of your back and begin again. After holding the contraction for five to ten seconds, relax completely, breathe in deeply and as you breathe out pull yourself forward slowly (holding the chest up as shown) until the required stretch is felt. Alternatively, you may reach further down the strap letting the back bend a little, and then restraighten by arching the back backwards and lifting the chest. Hold the final position for at least ten breaths. Repeat for the other leg.

In the **intermediate** assistance exercise, your partner supports whichever part of your back wants to bend first as you increase the pulling effort on the foot. If your partner places his or her hands on this most curved part of the back, straightening the back (and holding the final stretch position) will require far less effort. You will also be able to hold the final position longer. Ensure that you look forwards and try to keep the chest lifted up. These directions will help keep the back straight.

This ends the lower back rehabilitation section.

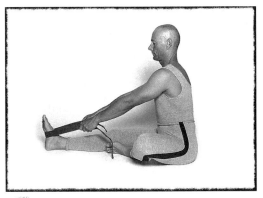

1   Solo version

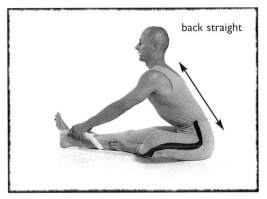

back straight

2

Notes

grasp strap at comfortable position

lift chest to straighten back

C–R: try to pull away from foot

go forwards to new position;
straighten back

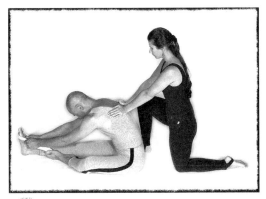

1   Partner version

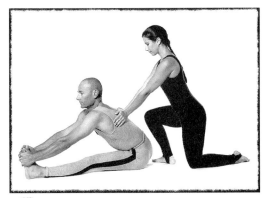

2   Advanced position foot grip

Notes (partner version)

partner supports roundest
part of back

lift the chest to straighten

C–R: while lifting chest,
press back

Breathe in; relax and restretch

MIDDLE BACK EXERCISES

12. Seated rotation

An effective rotation can be done using a chair. Look at the photographs. In the **easiest** version, sit across the seat to prevent the hips moving (bracing the side of the leg against the chair's back). Hold the chair back with an appropriate grip; the first image shows a thumb-up grip. Lift your chest up until your back feels straight (doing the exercise in front of a mirror is an excellent way to check your form). Use only your arms to turn your shoulders to one side until the desired stretch is felt, in the muscles along the spine in between the shoulder blades. Repeat for the other side.

The second photo shows an alternative grip, with the thumb down. This **intermediate** version allows a stretch to be felt in the muscles over the shoulder blades, and may be more effective for some people.

A partner **C–R version** of the exercise is the strongest, and for some people doing the partner version is the best way of learning where the stretch is supposed to be felt. Once you can feel this, the solo version described below becomes easier to do. Get into a moderate stretch position, which your partner supports. Notice that the partner's arms are straight. Most people are stronger and more stable this way, using the muscles of the waist and hips in preference to the muscles of the arms. The partner's hand and arm positions are shown in the photographs. You twist gently back against the restraint provided by the partner, who does not permit your shoulders to move at all from the stretch position. Do this for five to ten seconds. Stop pushing and take in a deep breath. As you breathe out, you use the arm holding the chair to take the shoulders further in the stretch direction. The partner holds you in the final position for ten breaths or so, or about thirty seconds. Repeat for the other side.

This is an excellent middle back stretch, and can be done anywhere there is a chair. It is excellent for those who work at keyboards, and can give great relief for people with *scoliosis*. This exercise can be a useful alternative to the lying rotations described earlier (exercises 3 and 4) for those people who cannot lie on one hip, or who have difficulty doing exercise on the floor.

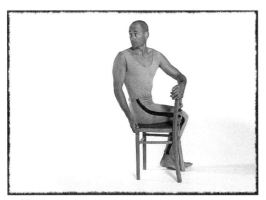

1 Easiest hand position (thumb up)

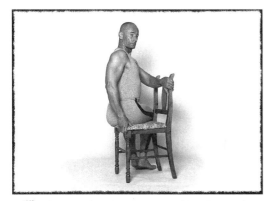

2 Intermediate hand position (thumb down)

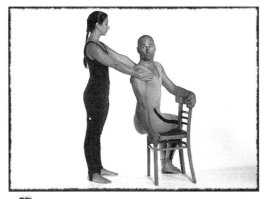

3 Push left shoulder back

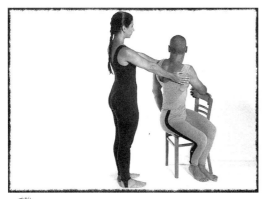

4 Going the other way

To do a solo **C–R version,** hold yourself in a gentle stretch position, and apply a light twisting force in the opposite direction using the muscles of the waist *against* the resistance of the arms, without letting the body move at all. Stop and take in a deep breath. Relax completely and, using your arms, rotate the shoulders further with respect to the hips. You must keep the back straight, and you must not force this technique. You may feel the major effects of this movement a little higher in the back than with the first version of the exercise. Precisely where you will feel the effects of any stretch depends on where you hold tension, which muscles you use for the C–R, and your proportions. Small adjustments in grip position (vertically) in this exercise can make major differences to where the stretch will be felt. Experiment to find the best stretch for you.

No advanced version of the exercise is shown, as you can get all the stretch you need using the the illustrated version—just go further around.

Notes

you must do the stretch
work yourself

keep both buttocks on the chair

lift chest to straighten back

C–R: can be done solo
or with partner

gently *pull* yourself into final
position

breathe normally

13. Upper back on all fours

This minor pose is often used to relax the lower and middle back muscles after backward bending, but is included here because it is a gentle and safe stretch in its own right. It is sometimes called the cat pose, because the shapes resemble the sort of stretches cats do upon awakening. I have added a contraction component to intensify the final position of the stretch, and a bend to the side (lateral flexion) to the normal spinal flexion movement.

In the **easiest** version, begin by kneeling on the floor. If the knees feel uncomfortable, kneel on a folded towel or the like—you cannot stretch properly if you are being distracted by discomfort anywhere in the body. Notice that the knees are under the hips, and the hands are slightly in front of the shoulders. Let the head slowly hang down under its own weight. When it has descended as far as it can, draw the chin into the chest. Feeling your weight evenly on hands and knees, slowly curl the body as shown. This requires the stomach (abdominal) muscles to be contracted. Take your time doing this, both to feel the stretch and to be aware of the location of the muscles being used.

To make this an **intermediate** stretch, in the final position use the muscles of the shoulders and arms to push the hands gently away from you as though you were trying to slide them away from you, while contracting the stomach muscles. This extra effort increases the stretch in the middle and, for some people, the upper back. Hold for five breaths in and out. Note that breathing will be difficult because the abdominal area is contracted and lung volume reduced. Return to the starting position.

Caution: for some people, the intermediate version of the exercise may make the stomach muscles cramp momentarily. If this happens, immediately arch the back backwards, and the muscles will relax. Muscles that are asked to do work in their contracted position (which is out of their normal working range of movement) will sometimes cramp. It is not a sign that there is anything wrong.

In the relaxed hands-and-knees position, slowly look around behind you, trying to see the heel of the foot on the side to which you are turning. Feel the contraction of the waist muscles on this side. This movement stretches the

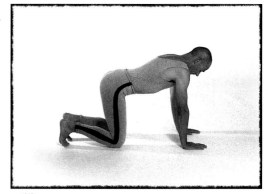

1 Kneel on something comfortable

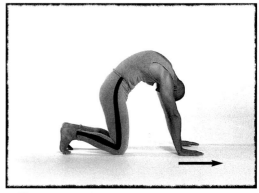

2 Gently push back on hands

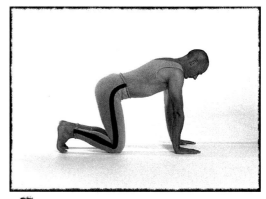

3 Relax

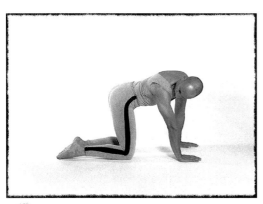

1 Look at one heel

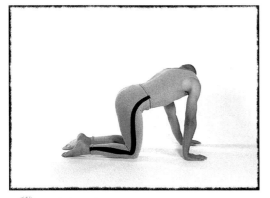

2 and the other

same muscle groups on the opposite side of the body. See if you can feel this. Repeat for the other side, and after holding the final position for a few seconds, briefly return to the first stretch position, and back to the starting position. The reason for returning briefly to the first stretch position is to relax the muscles which need to contract to produce the stretch position.

The advice to stretch a second time on the side you begin with is a general rule for the whole body. When stretching matched pairs of muscles which require the contraction of one of the pairs to produce the stretch in the other, you will benefit from repeating the first side's stretch briefly, to relax the last-used muscle group.

Notes

if your stomach muscles cramp, bend backwards gently

in the hands-and-knees position turn side-to-side slowly

14. Middle and upper back

This exercise stretches the middle to upper back, depending on your proportions. In addition to the *paravertebrals* (the muscles running alongside the spine), this exercise stretches *trapezius* and the *rhomboids*, and the movement is also one of the few solo stretches available for a pair of muscles that lift the shoulders (*levator scapulae*; these muscle groups are shown overleaf). As one end of levator scapulae attaches to the shoulder blade and the other to the side of the cervical spine, these muscles either elevate one or both shoulders or flex the neck to one side. Consequently, this exercise can also be used as an indirect neck stretching exercise.

Head placement is critical, both to avoid possible neck injury and to ensure that the stretch is felt in the correct muscles. Those who are stiff may find it difficult to get into the starting position; if so, try placing your forehead on the floor instead of the top of the head, the standard direction. If you still cannot get into position relatively easily, you may reattempt the movement after practicing other exercises (1, 12, 13 and 16, for example) for a while. Bulky people will find it difficult to get into the starting position, so use these other exercises instead.

In the **easiest** version, kneel down as shown. While supporting yourself with one arm, reach through the knees (notice that the knees are further apart than the ankles) and hold the foot of the same side with the indicated grip. Curl forwards and place the *top* of the head on the floor, and rest some of the body's weight on the head. This locates the shoulders with respect to the hips. Now reach through the knees with the other hand, and hold the other foot. If you cannot hold your feet, the final photograph shows an alternative grip using a strap. Ensure that the top of the head is resting on the floor. Breathe normally. Gripping the feet (or the strap) firmly, slowly and gently push the hips forwards. Because the hands are holding the feet, the middle and upper back are drawn into a forward curve, as in drawing a bow. Generally, this will not irritate the lower back if back pain is your problem—all of the stretch is felt higher in the back.

In the final position, breathe in and out for five breaths or so. Let the stretch go by letting the hips return to the start position. Take one hand off one foot, and place it in the support position. **Now breathe in, and hold your breath**

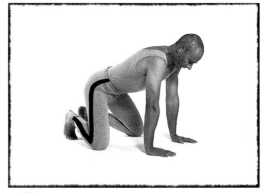

1   Knees far enough apart

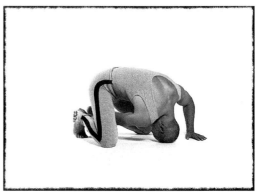

2   *Support* yourself to reach foot

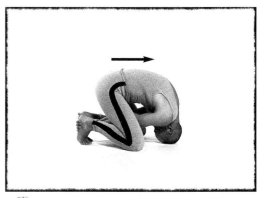

3   Push hips forwards

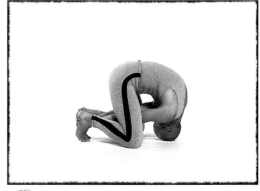

4   Final position

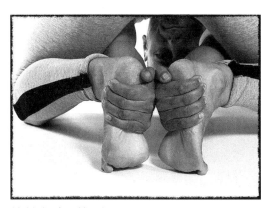
Hold the feet like this

while you use the support arm to lift yourself back to the beginning position. When there, resume normal breathing. Do not lift yourself up into the start position using the muscles of the back. As a general rule, when returning from any extended (stretched) position, use muscles other than the ones you have been stretching. You may move the main locus of the stretch further down to the middle of the back by holding the feet from outside the legs. Overleaf, Jennifer is demonstrating this alternative.

Two C–R stretches may be done. When in the stretch position (either version) try to shrug the shoulders while holding firmly onto the feet. This engages *levator scapulae* and consequently a stronger stretch will be felt in these muscles when you restretch. In the second C–R stretch, try to draw the shoulder blades together directly behind you while holding the feet firmly. Restretching will concentrate the effects in *trapezius* and the *rhomboids*. **If your stomach muscles cramp, come out of the pose and lift your arms up above your head.** Rest for a moment, and try the exercise again.

In combination with the neck exercises, exercises 13 & 14 will stretch the majority of muscles affected by office work, and keyboard work in particular. People with scoliosis should make this pair of exercises the cornerstone of their personal routine.

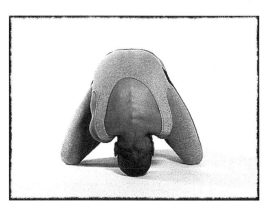
View of stretched middle and upper back muscles

Notes

rest head on blanket or cushion

top of head on floor (usual),
or forehead on floor
(to reduce stretch on neck)

don't hold your breath

push hips forwards gently

two C–Rs: shrug shoulders; restretch

pull shoulder blades together
behind you; restretch

*if stomach muscles cramp, come out of
pose and lift arms up above head*

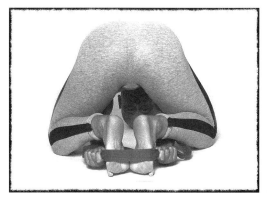
If you can't hold your feet, use a strap

In this version, you will need to have the knees a little closer together than the feet so that you can hold the feet without interference. All other directions for the exercise are the same as the version I am demonstrating. Try both versions, and use the one which gives you the best stretch sensation; the locus of effectiveness is strongly dependent on your proportion.

Levator scapulae

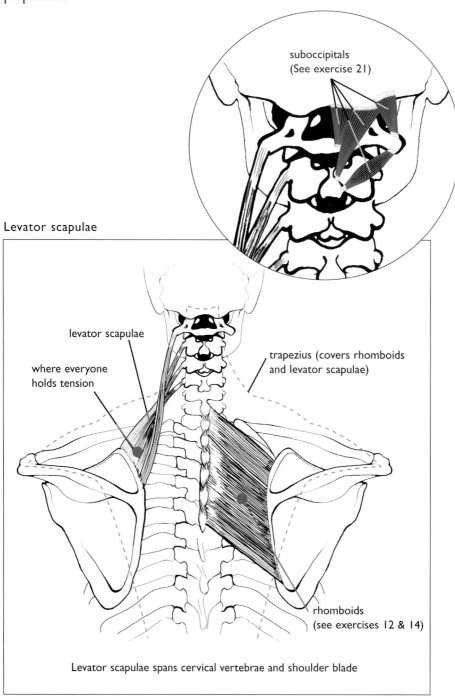

suboccipitals
(See exercise 21)

levator scapulae

where everyone
holds tension

trapezius (covers rhomboids
and levator scapulae)

rhomboids
(see exercises 12 & 14)

Levator scapulae spans cervical vertebrae and shoulder blade

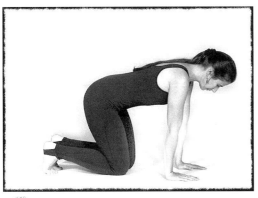

1 Support

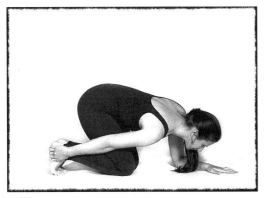

2 Reach

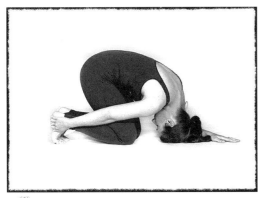

3 Top of head on floor

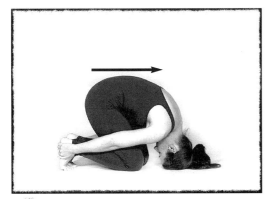

4 Push hips forwards

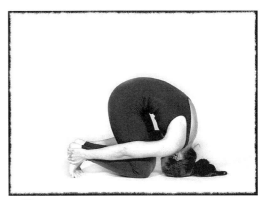

5 Final position

Notes

this version may suit your proportions

rest head on something comfortable

hold outside of feet to stretch lower down

a strap can be used here, too

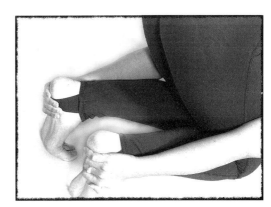

Hold feet from outside

NECK EXERCISES

15. Partner shoulder depress

Caution: those who suffer from any sort of lower back problem which renders them unduly sensitive to axial (longitudinal) compression of the spine should approach this exercise with care. Having said this, exercise 15 is the most popular of all the stretches presented in my classes. It makes everyone feel lighter, as though their cares have been lifted from their shoulders. In fact, as this movement stretches the muscles which hold the shoulders in their usual position, this is both literally and metaphorically true. This exercise is essential for people who spend much of their life at a keyboard or hunched over books.

As we become more tense, or as we are exposed to any frustrating experience, the shoulders move upward of their own accord. The muscles between the shoulders and neck become tight and painful. This reaction is universal, and over time, may lead to conditions such as "frozen shoulders." Tension in these muscles is nearly always present in people with neck pain, and the same tension invariably accompanies conditions such as Repetitive Strain Injury (now known as Occupational Overuse Syndrome). Tension in the *levator scapulae* and *scalene* muscles is always an accompanying phenomenon, the successful reduction of which alleviates much of the neck pain as well. Recall the last really relaxed person you saw: there would have been much open space between the ears and the shoulders, suggesting that (other things being equal) relaxed people carry their shoulders lower than those who are not. Angry people hold their shoulders up around their ears. This exercise will remove tension from this area.

The **easiest, C–R exercise** is suitable for everyone. Look at top photograph. We are using a bench to show the physical positions clearly, but you can use two strong (but nonsliding) chairs. Sit normally with your trunk against the back of the chair and your shoulders relaxed into their lowest position, and bottom well back into the chair. Your partner stands on a similarly strong chair (one which can support their whole weight), bends his or her knees slightly, inclines forward from the hips, and places straight arms (hands and fingers lightly cupping your shoulders) as shown. Once comfortable and secure in this position, the partner *leans forward from the waist* so that some of his or her weight is transferred evenly to both your shoulders. Doing the exercise in front of a mirror to check the level of the shoulders is helpful. If you are not using a chair, you will need to lean back slightly onto your partner's legs—otherwise when they lean on you, there will be a tendency for your upper back to bend forwards rather than the shoulders be pressed down.

Your partner *leans* weight on you (rather than *pushing* with the arm

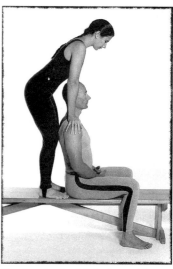

You lean back slightly for stability

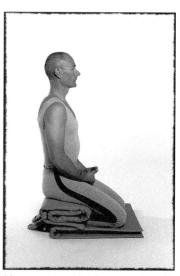

How to sit on the floor comfortably

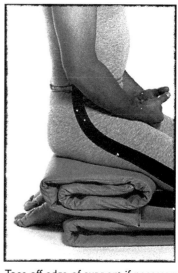

Toes off edge of support if necessary

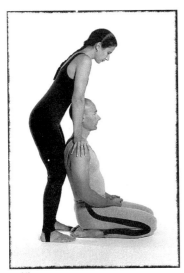

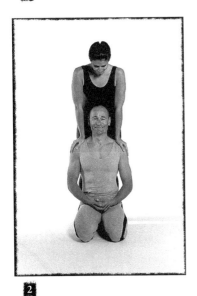

1 Lean back for support

2

Notes

muscles), so that you feel a stretch in the muscles mentioned. You need to hold your upper body straight while letting the shoulders be stretched. Once you have let yourself relax in the stretch position, ask your partner to hold the shoulders there; that is, to resist your attempts to lift the shoulders. When your partner is ready, slowly lift your shoulders moderately strongly (the partner resisting all the while) for ten seconds or so. Your partner must not allow the shoulders to move. *If you can move your shoulders, you are lifting too much, or your partner is not leaning enough weight.* When you have completed the contraction phase, warn your partner that you are about to stop lifting, and do so. (The warning is so they do not end up on top of you!)

Take a deep breath and, letting the shoulders relax completely, ask the partner to lean on you once more. You will find that the shoulders drop quite dramatically, giving you a pleasing stretch in the area between the neck and the shoulders. Repeat the lifting–holding–relaxing sequence up to a total of three times—beyond this, any additional effect is usually negligible. To finish, the partner removes their weight, and you lift the shoulders up and down, letting them sink down to their new relaxed position.

Notice from the photographs that the exercise may be done from the kneeling seated position if this is comfortable for you. No strain should be felt in the knees in this position. A firm pillow or similar object placed between the bottom and the heels will help the legs feel comfortable. If there is too much stretch in the insteps (from being stretched backward), sit across a cushion in such as way as to relieve the instep and toes; a second cushion goes between the bottom and the heels as before. In the kneeling version, you should lean backwards against your partner's knees for support, but do not exaggerate this. All other directions are the same as the chair version.

See exercises 14, 17 & 18 for further stretches for *levator scapulae* and 19 for the *scalene* muscles.

16. Chin to chest

The purpose of this exercise is to stretch the muscles controlling the movement of the head backwards (the movement called *extension*). The head itself tilts on the spine (the *cervical vertebrae;* the first two are involved in this movement, mainly) and the cervical spine itself bends forwards in relation to the rest of the body, in the movement called *flexion*. This distinction is made because two C–R stretches are offered that separately stretch the muscles under the back of the skull (the *suboccipitals*) and the muscles that extend the neck and the head. When doing the second part of the exercise, it is possible to feel the stretch in only one small local area along the back of the neck even though the whole neck appears to be curved. This may only mean that this is the place where you hold the most tension.

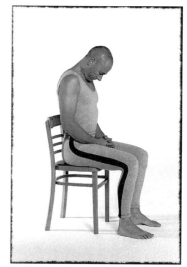

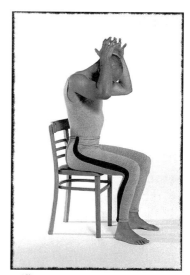

1 Easiest

In the **easiest** version, you incline the head forward, trying to divide the movement into tilting of the head and bending the neck itself. When you have reached a position of stretch, hold it for a few breaths in and out, letting the tension go. When you have relaxed sufficiently, place your clasped hands on what is now the top of your head (somewhere behind where the top normally is) and gently let the weight of the arms rest on the head. Let this weight come onto the back of the neck slowly, so that if the stretch becomes too strong you can remove the arms' weight before you hurt yourself. As the weight is felt, the head will incline further towards the chest. Feel the stretch, visualizing the tension leaving the body with each breath out, and try to feel the stretch over as much of the back of the neck as possible. ("Visualising" means trying to see clearly in your mind that the tension you feel is moving out of the place you feel it, and is leaving the body with each breath out.) Stay in the final position for five to ten breaths. To come out of the stretch, remove the hands from the top of the head, slowly lift the head to the neutral position, and rest.

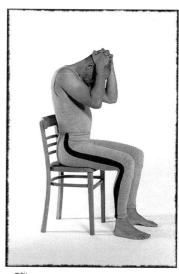

2

There are **two C–R stretches**, both requiring care. On a general note, we have found that neck muscles do not require long contractions to help them relax. Until this point in the book, we have been using contractions of five to ten seconds' duration. With neck muscles, *two to five seconds* will be sufficient, and in the relax phase, two to five breaths at normal speed should be sufficient. Of course, you may increase either of these recommended times if you feel that you need longer. Once the neck muscles are accustomed to the weight of the arms on the back of the neck, very gently try to tilt the head backwards, by *trying to lift the chin* in the stretch position (rather than pushing the whole head backwards). On a breath out, restretch carefully. This version activates the small muscles under the back of the skull (the *suboccipitals*). Holding tension in these muscles can lead to the familiar "tension headaches." **A**

3

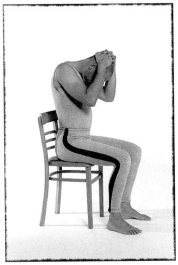

4 Stretch neck forwards gently

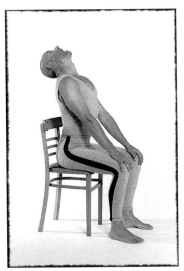

5 Tilt back with mouth open

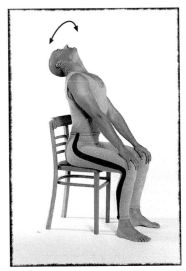

6 Incline head slightly left and right

stronger stretch for each set of *suboccipitals* will be found in exercise 21.

In the **second C–R stretch**, very gently push the head back against the resistance of your hands for a few seconds. Remove the hands for a second or two, then replace them. While breathing out, restretch extremely cautiously. Hold the final position for five breaths.

After stretching forwards, it is good to stretch backwards briefly and gently, and to restretch forwards for a moment. This makes the neck feel most comfortable (in contrast with only stretching forwards). The safest way, after you have come back to the starting position, is to *open the mouth wide*, keep the shoulders relaxed, and slowly tilt the head backwards as far as you can. When in the final stretch position, gently close the teeth together. Keep the back straight—do not confuse leaning backwards with stretching the neck. Closing the teeth after you have moved the head backwards helps concentrate the stretch in the muscles and skin at the front of the throat, and reduces any uncomfortable compression in the joints of the spine at the back of the neck.

Once in the final stretch position, you may incline the head gently to one side. So doing will stretch the front neck muscles on the side of the neck you are stretching away from. Hold the new position for a breath or two, slowly incline the head to the other side, and hold for the same duration. Check to see if there are any left-right differences. **Always follow a backwards neck bending movement with a gentle forwards stretch**, for a few seconds. This will relieve any discomfort in the muscles in the back of the neck, which in some people tend to tighten when the head is taken backwards.

Notes

move into stretch cautiously

two C–Rs: press head back, restretch

and lift chin forwards away from body while holding head

restretch on breath in and out

17. Neck side bend

Much neck pain is felt in the side of the neck, and most often on the dominant arm side, indicated by left or right handedness. This exercise will stretch some of the muscles involved, and is a complement to the exercise 15 (the one where your partner leans down on your shoulders). As you will know (and certainly will see if you watch yourself), bending the neck to the side is usually achieved in part by lifting the shoulder we are stretching away from and by inclining the whole body. Knowing this, we can concentrate the stretch in the side neck muscles by restraining the shoulder we are stretching away from.

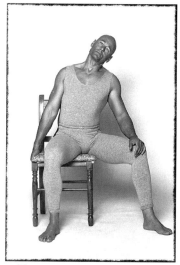

1 Easiest

In the **easiest version**, you hold the seat of the chair with one hand. Keep the back straight (as seen from the side). If you have a tendency to be a little hunched over, breathe in and lift the chest before you begin and hold the body straight during the exercise. Watch yourself—as you lift the chest, the upper back straightens. Ensure that the head is over the shoulders (as it might be seen from the side). Now, incline the head to the side, away from the restrained shoulder. Here too we are trying to make the whole neck curve to the side, as well as tilting the head on the neck. Avoid doing only one or the other. Do not rotate the head or bend the neck forwards. The movement ideally occurs in one plane only, the vertical plane going through both shoulders. The stretch will be felt in the side of the neck, anywhere from the shoulder to the ear, and perhaps in the arm holding the chair.

The **intermediate** version requires care. When in the fully-stretched position, and after having held this position for three or four breaths in and out, reach up with the free hand and place two fingers on the side of the head above the ear as shown. Very gently press these fingers onto the side of the head to increase the stretch fractionally. Hold the final position for a few breaths. This must be done extremely sensitively. Err on the side of not using enough pressure.

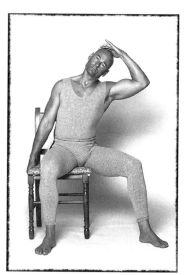

2 Intermediate

Alternatively, you can use **two C–R stretches** to enhance the stretch effects, if you are careful. Rather than using the fingers to stretch the neck further, place the two fingers on the head as before, but this time use the fingers only as a barrier to press against. In the **first contraction**, try to shrug the shoulder of the restraining hand for a few seconds. Stop shrugging, take a breath in, and on a breath out lean the body further away from the restraining hand. This will stretch you above the shoulder. For the **second C–R**, gently press the head back against your fingers for a few seconds. Stop pressing, and take the fingers from the head for a second or two. Replace the fingers, and while breathing out, very gently restretch. Hold the final position for five breaths in and out. Repeat for the other side. These C–R stretches may be used singly or together.

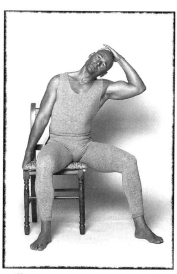

3 Final position

Notes

leg out to side for stability

move head *sideways* only

hang from arm

Two C–Rs: shrug shoulder
of arm holding chair, and

press head gently against
two fingers

cautiously restretch after breath
in and out

Front and side neck muscles

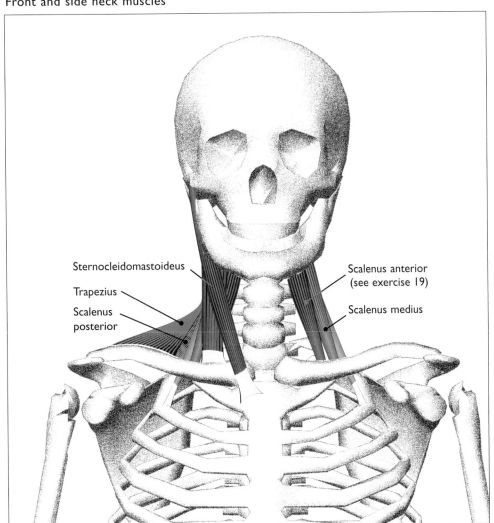

Sternocleidomastoideus

Trapezius

Scalenus
posterior

Scalenus anterior
(see exercise 19)

Scalenus medius

18. Neck forward and side bend

This is the most important neck exercise. It can relieve neck pain (particularly behind the ear or down to above the shoulder blade), mandibular pain, and combined with exercise 19, can be very effective for referred pain in the shoulders, arms or hands. Even if you do not have any of these problems, this exercise is likely to have the strongest effect on both the feeling of comfort in your neck and your feeling of well-being. This is likely the result of relieving some of the tension that most people carry in their necks and which seems to most directly affect mood. It is the first exercise I use in my *Practical* **Stress Management** workshops. I have yet to meet a manager who does not hold tension in these muscles, and who does not express amazement at the difference in mood that results from spending a minute or so doing the movement. Everyone will know which muscles are affected without looking at an illustration: they are the muscles that everyone wants massaged! This is the strongest stretch for *levator scapulae* (refer back to the illustration on page 78).

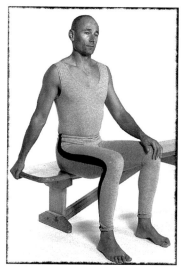
1 Hand *behind* hip

The movement is a combination of forward and side bending (flexion and lateral flexion), and may be altered with a small rotation, depending on where you wish to feel the stretch. The directions are complicated, but no other neck stretch will leave the neck feeling as good as this one will. Examine the photographs carefully before trying it for the first time, and note the directions of the assistance movements.

In the **easiest** version, begin as with exercise 17, restraining the shoulder by holding onto the seat of the chair, but with the hand a little further behind the hip joint than before. Experiment with placement—five to six inches behind the hip is a good starting position. Lean both to the side and slightly forwards. This will mean *directly away* from the hand restraining the shoulder. Let the chin go all the way forwards onto the chest, pause, then take the head to the side using your neck muscles. At this point, the head will be directly opposite the restraining hand, meaning that the neck is both flexed and laterally flexed. You may feel the stretch anywhere from the ear down to the shoulder, and anyone with overuse injuries is likely to feel the stretch in the arm as well.

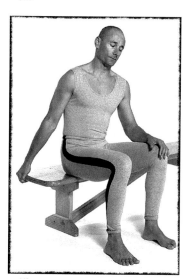
2 Lean away from hand

To make this an **intermediate** stretch, reach up with the other hand, and place two fingers on the head, opposite the restraining hand. To focus the stretch exactly where you need it, try turning the head slightly to the side of the restraining hand. You can alter the precise locus of the stretch by making very small adjustments to either the position of the head in relation to your body, or by turning the head very slightly left or right.

Once the ideal spot is located, **two C–R stretches** may be used. First, shrug the shoulder of the hand holding the support. Stop shrugging, breathe in, and restretch *by leaning further away from the hand holding the*

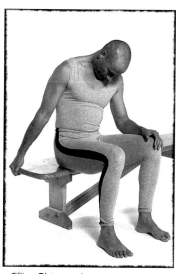
3 Chin to chest

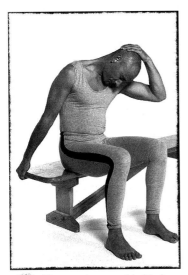

4 Fingers above and behind ear

chair. Take the head and body further into the stretch together. The main effect will be to stretch the neck muscles where they join the body or the shoulder.

In the **second C–R,** once in the position achieved by the first C–R, press the head very gently back against the fingers using the muscles you feel the stretch in. Again stop pressing. To restretch, use the fingers on the head *to take the head closer to the chest,* and **while holding the head in its forward-most position,** gently take the head further to the side. Hold the final position for five breaths. Repeat for the other side. The most common mistake is not to hold the head forwards as it is taken to the side. If you do not hold the head forwards, much of the potential stretch effect will be lost. Most of the stretch effect of this second version will be felt in the muscles of the side of the neck itself.

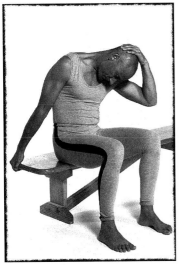

5 *Forwards* before sideways

Notes

move into stretch position cautiously

two C–Rs: shrug shoulder of arm holding chair,

and press head gently against two fingers

re-stretch after breath, very softly

turning head to change stretch

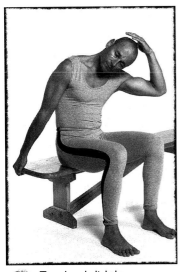

6 Turn head slightly,

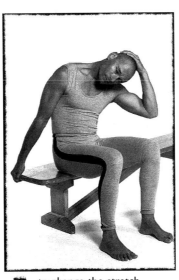

7 to change the stretch

19. Neck backward and side bend

This exercise is technically difficult to practice, but for certain types of neck and arm problems, there is no better remedy. The muscles stretched in this are the *scalenes*, which are muscles commonly implicated in entrapment of the nerves of the arm (the *brachial plexus*). Refer to the illustration on the facing page. You will notice that the nerves of the arm pass in between the front and middle scalenes, and pass over the first rib. If these muscles are tight or in spasm, or if the first rib has been displaced slightly vertically (as may happen in a car accident, for example), then these structures can put pressure on the nerves. This may lead to Thoracic Outlet Compression Syndrome (TOCS, or sometimes TOS). Sufferers report a wide variety of symptoms, ranging from referred pain into the front of the chest, side or back of the shoulder, pain in the forearm muscles (especially the front, near the crook of the elbow), reduced grip strength, and loss of feeling or tingling in the fingers— usually the thumb and first finger, but occasionally the others, too. The difficulty in practicing the exercise arises because bending the neck back and to the side can cause cramping in the muscles of the back of the neck, on the side that you are bending towards.

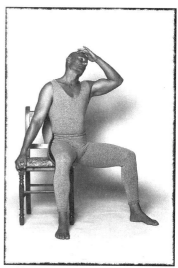

3 Turn head to find right angle

Recall that to stretch the muscles at the side of the neck (exercise 17) we needed to lean directly away from a hand placed *opposite* the hip, and that to stretch the muscles at the back and side of the neck, we needed to place the hand *behind* the hip (exercise 18). To stretch the *scalenes* (located at the front and side of the neck) a similar approach to the two previous exercises is used. Hold the support about five to six inches *in front of* the hip joint, and lean the head *back and to the side*, again directly away from the hand. In the **easiest** version, lean away from the hand until a stretch is felt in the muscles at the front and side of the neck, on the side you are stretching away from. Hold this position for a few breaths in and out. To come out of the position, *bring the head back to the neutral position*, and only then use the arm to return the body to the starting position.

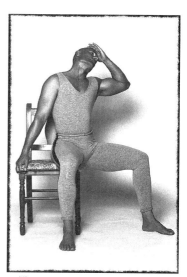

2 Hold head for both C–Rs

Caution: bending the neck back and to the sides may cause other muscles at the back of your neck to cramp (go into spasm). If this happens, immediately bend your head and neck in the *opposite* direction. If you suspect that this may occur, review exercise 18 (which stretches the neck in the opposite direction) before you begin.

Two C–R stretches are used as before. Slightly turning the head away from, or towards, the restraining hand will locate the most effective stretch positions. For the **first C–R**, place two fingers of the free hand against the temple, opposite the restraining hand as a barrier to head movement. Gently shrug the shoulder of the arm holding the chair, and restretch by leaning the body a little further into the stretch direction. In

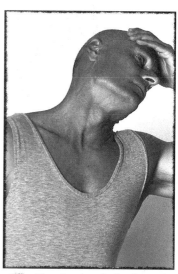

1 Easiest

hang from arm

Two C–Rs: shrug the shoulder,
restretch, and

press temple gently
against fingers

very cautiously restretch after
breath in and out

use wall behind you to limit
movement if necessary

the **second C–R**, hold the new stretch position gained by the first C–R, and very gently press the head against the fingers holding your temple. This will directly activate the *scalenes*. After pressing for a few seconds, pause, and after a breath out very cautiously restretch. Hold the final position for a few breaths in and out, and return to the starting position by releasing the head, and only then use the supporting arm to bring the body back.

Possible entrapment of nerves by scalene muscles

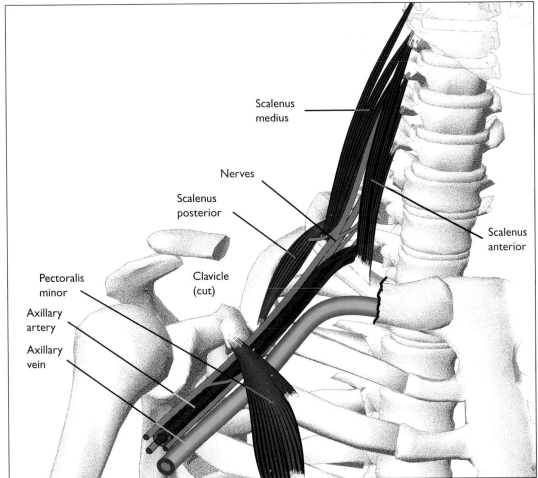

It may be that the exercise as described is too strong in its effects on the *scalenes* for some people. If so, you may care to try a modified version of the exercise, which uses the support provided by the edge of a mattress. Look at the last photograph. Here, I am using a few mats to simulate a suitable surface. Holding your head in a neutral position (neither forwards nor backwards), slide yourself to the edge, letting the head go over, but with the mattress fully supporting the back of the skull and the whole of the neck. The first time you try this, only let the top half of your head go over the edge. Very slowly, let the weight of your head compress the edge of the mattress, so that the neck is gently bent backwards until sufficient stretch is felt in the front of the neck. While still holding your head, cautiously turn the head to one side to stretch the *scalenes* more directly. Only let the head go backwards and around to the extent of feeling the desired stretch. Rotate the head to the other side and stretch, and return to the center. Use your arms to lift your head back to a comfortable position and sit up.

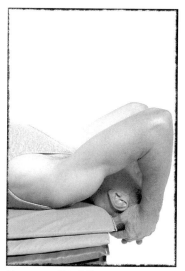

Ensure neck is fully supported

Notes

do not let your head
go over too far

arms support head at all times

once in position, very slowly
turn head until stretch is felt

use arms to return to start
position

20. Neck rotation

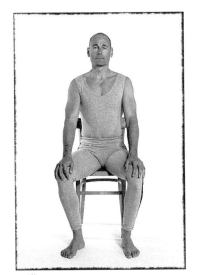

1

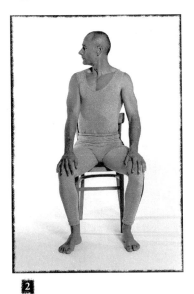

2

This stretch demonstrates how much your normal pattern of movement constrains your actively available flexibility. Look at the photograph. Sit squarely on the chair, with your weight evenly on both bottom bones, leaning neither forwards nor backwards, with your back straight and body relaxed. Slowly turn your head to one side without inclining it forwards and without tilting it to the side. The movement is pure rotation. Turn the head as far as you can, and when it will go no further, hold the final position. Pause, take a deep breath in, and as you exhale, *try to turn the head further*. Considerable extra movement will be achieved with the second effort. Hold the final position for a few breaths in and out, and feel the muscles being stretched (at the side of the neck you are stretching away from) and the muscles you are using (at the side of the neck and between the neck and the shoulder you are stretching towards). Repeat for the other side, but finish with a brief rotation towards the side you stretched first, to release the muscles you used to achieve the second movement.

The interesting aspect of this exercise is that even if you know that you will be able to turn further with a second effort, the head will not go beyond a certain position when you turn it the first time. A second effort usually produces further movement, however. This suggests that flexibility is a phenomenon deriving both from structure and patterns of use; in other words, a neuromuscular phenomenon. With respect to any left-right difference found in this exercise, a question to ask may be, "Over which shoulder do you look as you back your car out of the garage each day?"

No contractions or assistance movements are required to improve rotation. The great bulk of the neck muscles are involved in this movement, either by contracting to achieve the rotation or the opposite groups being stretched by the movement, or by doing isometric work so that particular muscles can produce the whole movement. Accordingly, this exercise allows you to feel where limitations may exist in your movement. Turning the head in this way against the resistance of the neck's own muscles is also an excellent strengthening exercise.

Notes

only *turn* your head; do not incline or tilt

turn as far as you can, and pause

after a breath in and out, turn further

hold final position for a few breaths

21. Chin-to-chest variations

This exercise allows you to stretch the muscles at the back and side of the neck, but unlike exercise 16 (from which these movements are derived) only half of the neck is stretched at a time. This permits comparison of left and right, and allows you to concentrate on a problem area specifically. Additionally, the second part of this exercise is the best *suboccipitals* exercise we have found. Refer back to page 78 for details.

Both versions of this exercise begin with the same starting position. In the **easiest** version, sit up straight, towards the front of the chair, with your feet underneath your knees for stability. Let the chin move forward towards the center of the chest, or as far as it will go. Clasp your hands together and place them on what is now the top of the head. Allow the weight of the completely relaxed arms to rest on the head, if you can. Notice that the elbows hang down; they are not held out to the sides—if they are, you are not permitting the full weight of the arms to do its job. In the first movement, having assumed the starting position and moved into the stretched position, you *slowly rotate at the waist*. Rotate until your elbows are above either side of one knee, or until you feel a stretch down the side of the neck you are stretching away from. This should be felt all the way to the top of the shoulder blade. Hold this second position for a few breaths. This movement is a strong stretch for *levator scapulae* in particular. A **C–R stretch** may be achieved by gently pressing the head back against the hands in the rotated position, and restretching. A **second C–R stretch** is achieved by trying to lift the chin forwards, away from the chest.

The **intermediate** movement achieves an additional stretch by letting the hips roll *backwards* while holding the previous stretch. This curving of the spine moves the stretch further down the back, and increases the stretch in the previously mentioned muscles. Hold the final position for a few breaths. A **C–R stretch** may be added here too, by pressing the head back from the final position, and restretching after a breath out. Remove the hands from the head, and *only then* return to the starting position. The reason for this direction is that because you are stretching you are out of the normal working range of the muscles. Potentially, the neck muscles could be strained if they are used to lift both the weight of the arms and the head at the same time. Repeat for the other side of the neck.

A **variation** of the exercise begins the same way, except that you may wish to have the knees a little further apart for sideways stability. After assuming the first stretch position, *incline the whole upper body to one side*, as close to purely sideways (that is, the plane of the shoulders) as you can. Notice that as the body inclines sideways, the lower arm drops away from the head while the other rests on it. If this does not happen, the

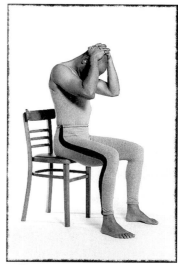

1 Easiest (end position, ex. 16)

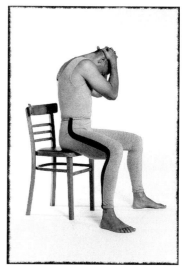

2 Rotate at waist

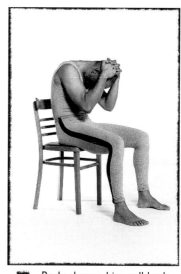

3 Body slumps, hips roll back

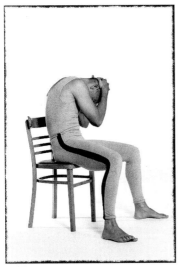

4 Intermediate

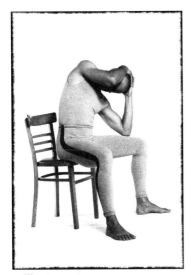

5 Second variation

Notes (opposite)

rotate *only* for the easiest version

hips roll back (intermediate)

two C–Rs: press head back against hands; lift chin forwards

weight of the top arm will not be felt properly. The stretch will be felt in the side of the neck you are stretching away from, but closer to the ear than the previous exercise. After holding the final position for a few breaths in and out, remove the arms from the head, and only then return to the start position. Repeat for the other side. The **C–R version** (which mainly stretches the *suboccipital* muscles on the side you are inclining away from) is very strong, so make the contraction element gentle. In the stretch position, press the head *backwards*, trying to use the muscles closest to the bottom of the skull. Breathe and restretch as usual.

You will see that exercises 16, 17, 18 and 21 can be done together. If you finish by taking the head backwards (last part of exercise 16) and add exercise 20 to end the session, doing all the exercises with C–Rs and variations will take but a few minutes. Any of these can be used in the office situation for loosening a tight muscle, as they all require a chair. The exercises may be done without a chair if you wish, by sitting on the hand used to restrain the shoulder. I would not usually include the *scalene* exercise (19) in a regular routine (unless you suffer the problems described in that exercise's introduction), but it may be used from time to time to check the tension in these key muscles. I have shown the exercises in idealized forms for teaching convenience, but there are many intermediate positions between stretching forwards and sideways where you might find an excellent stretch. Exercise 18 may be used at the keyboard any time for immediate relief of tension in the neck and shoulder area. This completes the rehabilitation neck stretching exercises.

Notes

incline *sideways* from waist for second variation

C–R: press head back against hands

restretch after breath out after all C–Rs

let head go before sitting up (both positions)

PREVENTION

The exercises in this chapter are *not* to be used by anyone suffering neck or back pain. They are to be used when the rehabilitation exercises have been successful. These are strong stretching and strengthening movements and are potentially dangerous. You must practice these movements with caution. If any sign of your previous problem arises, stop doing the new exercises for a week and return to the rehabilitation exercises from the previous chapter.

In comparison to chapter two, these exercises use a more "whole body" approach; that is, rather than targeting a single area, these exercises involve more than one joint and accordingly more than one muscle group. Precisely where you feel the stretch in any particular exercise will depend on lifestyle, proportion, and past problems. Experiment with small variations in positions to move the effect of any stretch to particular places.

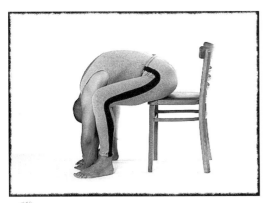

2 Lift head, try to straighten back

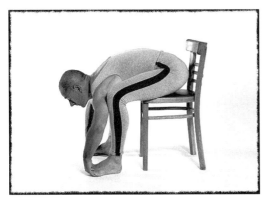

1 End position exercise I

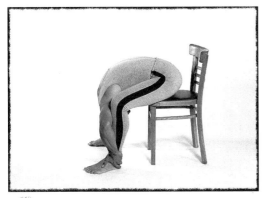

3 Use arm strength only to stretch

Notes

pull forwards gently to stretch

C–R: try to *straighten* back

after breath, pull on ankles
to restretch

22. Advanced forward bend

The first photograph shows the final position of exercise 1, seated forward bend. Reread the directions if you are not sure of precisely how to get into and out of the position.

This version employs a **C–R stretch** for the muscles of the lumbar spine primarily, and also for the buttock, hamstring , and inner thigh muscles. Assuming that you are in a stretched position, hold onto your feet as shown (or your ankles, if you cannot reach your feet). The contraction is achieved by using the back muscles (primarily) *in a back-straightening movement* to try gently to pull the hands away from the feet, by lifting the head and trying to arch the back backwards. This will be an isometric contraction. If you were to hold your back in the curved (starting) position as you try to lift the hands away from the feet, the main effect may be felt in the secondary muscles mentioned above. However, if you try to pull the hands away from the feet by using a back straightening effort, the main stretch effects will be felt in the muscles of the lumbar spine. Recall that a C–R effect is mainly felt in the muscles used to perform a contraction. To this end, before you try to pull the hands away from the feet, breathe out, lift the head away from the chest and take a half breath in. Contract the back muscles against the resistance of both your arms and the combined buttock, hamstring , and inner thigh muscles, holding the contraction for a count of between three and five. Describing the action is far more complicated than doing it, as you'll see.

This straightening effort must be small—a small, slowly and gently applied effort. Stop contracting, pause, and breathe in deeply. As you breathe out, let the head sink forwards again and very gently use the strength of your arms to restretch the back muscles. Notice where the stretch is.

You can move the focus of the stretch up and down the back by adjusting the force you apply. If you pull yourself more forwards, the stretch will move lower down the back; if you pull yourself more to the floor, the stretch will move higher up the back. Remain in the final position for five breaths in and out. Come out of the position using the arms.

For the easiest and intermediate versions of this exercise, see exercise 1.

23. Advanced forward and side bend

The following exercises are **advanced** versions of exercise 10 and exercise 11. This combination will provide strong stretches for the majority of the lower back muscles, especially the *oblique* group, *quadratus lumborum, erector spinae* and *latissimus dorsi*, and the *hamstring* group in turn. Following this, a **second advanced** version practiced with the legs apart combines these aspects, and adds a stretch for the *adductors* (the muscles of the inner thighs which pull the legs together). A strap may be used to hold the foot in either exercise.

To get into the start position, fold one leg, and bring it into the body as shown. The hips should be aligned square with the straight leg. Lean towards the leg, and hold the big toe with thumb and index finger, with the palm turned up. Pull on the big toe to bend the elbow, and lean further to the side to put the elbow on or close to the floor. Press the elbow against the inside of the leg (this brings the bottom shoulder closer to the center line of the body), and holding the shoulder in position roll the top shoulder back as far as you can. Thus, the first movement is a side bend and rotation of the trunk. Take a breath in, and as you breathe out reach the top arm out as far as you can, and grasp the foot. Now, in addition to the powerful side bend, the whole *latissimus dorsi* muscle on the top side of the body is stretched. The degree of stretch is controlled by how much you pull with the top arm.

A **C–R stretch** may be used here. When in the final position and after having stretched for half a minute or so, use the muscles of the waist to *try* to pull yourself away from your foot. All the trunk muscles described above will be involved in this effort; accordingly, when you restretch the effect in these muscles will be heightened. Hold the final position for a minute or more.

This prepares us for the next part of the exercise, an isolation movement for the hamstring muscles of one leg. Look at photograph 5. Turn to face one leg, holding the shoulders level with the floor. Link your hands and grasp one foot, keeping the center of your body over the leg. Reach down to the foot so that the back bends a little. The stretch in the hamstrings is achieved by holding the foot with straight arms, and slowly straightening the back. The direction to "hold with straight arms" is to ensure that any

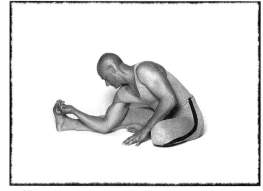

1 Press elbow back to bring shoulder forwards

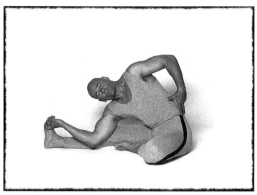

2 Roll top shoulder back

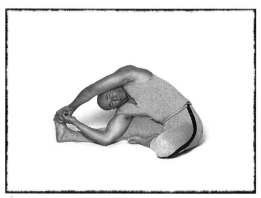

3 Hold foot with top arm to stretch side

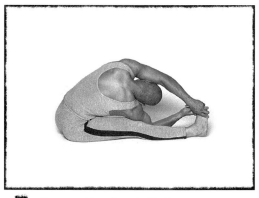

4 Same position, from behind

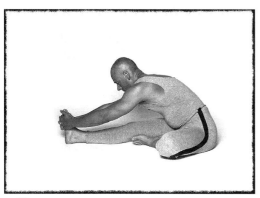

1 Grasp foot firmly

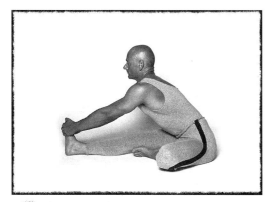

2 Straighten back

Notes (above)

hold foot with both hands

C–R: lift chest and try to pull
away from foot

Notes (opposite)

hold big toe with palm-up grip

press elbow to inside of leg

roll top shoulder back

reach top arm out; hold foot

C–R: use waist muscles to try to
pull away from foot

straightening action of the back is transferred to the hamstring muscles at the back of the leg, and also because it is easier to hold the final stretch position for longer if the *biceps brachii* muscles (the front of the upper arm) are not being used. The straightening action is also an isometric strengthening exercise for the back muscles running the whole length of the spine. Do not compromise straightness of the back to get the body closer to the leg. Hold the final position for ten breaths in and out. An even longer stay in this position yields good results—the hamstrings are powerful muscles, often very tight, and respond well to a long stretch.

To use a **C–R stretch,** lift the chest up to exaggerate the straightness of the back, and at the same time try to pull your hands away from the foot. If you are doing this correctly, the only place you will feel anything is in the hamstring muscles of the straight leg as they do the work of trying to take the body away from the leg—if you feel a strong effect in the back, you can be certain that (despite your best efforts!) it is not being held straight. Relax, pull yourself forwards with the arms letting the back bend a little, and re-straighten the back. Hold the final position for at least a minute; and more time spent in the pose will have an even stronger effect on the hamstrings .

The legs-apart version of this exercise is a major pose in Yoga and all the oriental exercise forms, and many health-giving benefits are ascribed to it, mainly to do with liver function. The exercise is fundamental to gymnastics and dance. To get into position, sit on the floor with your legs outstretched and as far apart as you can reasonably manage. If you cannot sit as shown with a straight back (probably due to tight hamstrings or adductors) you are not ready to do this pose, and are well advised to spend more time on the earlier exercises (especially 10 and 11). Lean over one leg, and hold the big toe as shown. Bend the arm and place the elbow in front of the leg you are leaning over, as in the version described above. Press the outside of this arm against the inside of the leg, to bring the shoulder at least above, and preferably inside, the line of the leg. Use the elbow in this position as a brace, around which to rotate your other shoulder as far back as possible (ideally, until it is vertical, as shown). You may feel the stretch in the side of the waist, above the hip, and along the back of (and perhaps even inside) the leg you are stretching over. If you have just practiced the version described above, you may be surprised to find that the legs-apart version is *less* of a stretch for the trunk muscles. This is because if you have any flexibility in the hamstring muscles at all, the *ischial tuberosity* (the bottom bone) of the opposite hip lifts slightly from the floor as you lean to the side (if you look carefully at photograph 3, you will see that my left hip is off the floor), and the stretch to the side is reduced by this amount. So, if you want a maximum waist or lower back stretch, the simpler-appearing one-leg version above is significantly stronger.

The **C–R stretch** version is essentially the same as for the one-leg version.

When you turn to one leg to stretch the hamstring group, you will notice the major difference between the single-leg and legs-apart versions. The wider you have your legs apart, the more you have to rotate the trunk to be able to face the leg. So, instead of bending forwards with a straight back and the shoulders aligned with the hips as in the single-leg version, now a considerable rotation is added to the straight back, stretching the muscles in a different way. Initially, when you reach for the foot, hold it with one hand only (see photograph 7) and lift the chest and straighten the back. The center of the body should be over the leg. Doing the exercise in this step-by-step way will help you to become

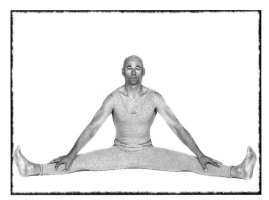

1 Legs as wide apart as possible

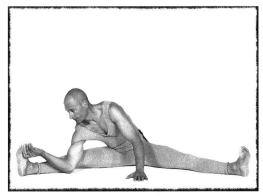

2 Elbow inside leg as pivot

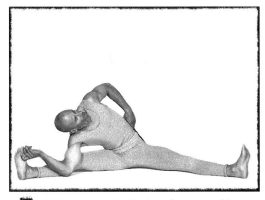

3 Roll top shoulder back as far as possible

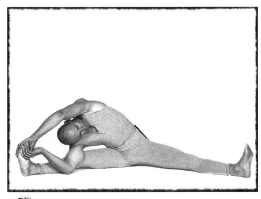

4 Top hand holds foot to stretch side

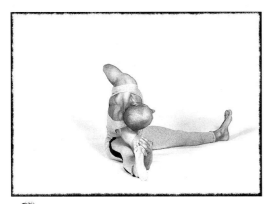

5   Photo 3 position from side

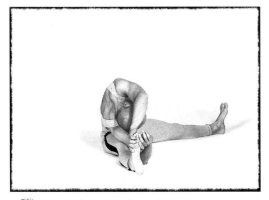

6   Photo 4 position from side

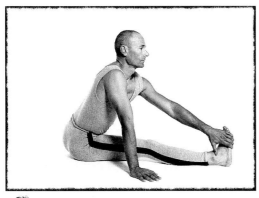

7   To stretch the hamstrings

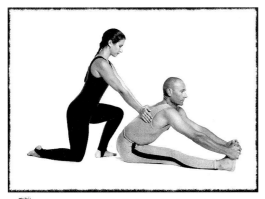

8   A partner can help keep back straight

aware of the proper alignment. Then reach for the foot with both hands as before and use the strength of the arms to pull the body in the direction of the leg. A partner can help with the stretch by helping you to hold your back straight.

The **C–R stretch** version is essentially the same as before, making sure that you emphasize the chest-lifting aspect as you pull back. When the contraction is completed, breathe in, relax the whole body except for the hands holding the foot, and pull the body closer to the foot. Hold the final position for at least a minute, concentrating on breathing in and out in a relaxed fashion. Do the other side. When you know which is the tighter side, begin the next practice session with this side, do the looser side, and do a final stretch for the first side. A partner can assist by placing his or her hands on the roundest part of your back to help you keep it straight, and by being a barrier to push against.

Notes

hold foot with *palm-up* grip
(on foot or strap)

roll shoulder back as far
as you can

breathe out, and reach
to the side

hold for 5–10 breaths

face leg; hold foot with
opposite hand

keep back straight

hold for 5–10 breaths

C–Rs can be done in
both positions

24. Advanced rotation

Before attempting this exercise, it may be useful to practice a suitable version of exercise 2 as a warmup. Exercise 24 is an extremely powerful trunk rotation movement whose effects can be subtly altered by how you position the body between the legs.

I will describe the seated version. Look at photograph 1. I have leaned forwards as in exercise 1, and grasped my right ankle with my left hand. Notice that my body is positioned *in between* my knees; this gives the most symmetrical stretch to the whole of the trunk. Positioning of the body is done by the degree of bend in the bottom arm. To apply the rotation, place the other hand on the knee of the same leg and press its shoulder back until the desired stretch is felt. To increase the stretch, pull on the hand holding the ankle, and push on the top arm.

A **C–R version** is easily done. While holding yourself in the stretch position firmly with both arms, try to twist the shoulders back in the opposite direction using the trunk muscles for five to ten seconds. After the contraction, without releasing the position, breathe in and out, and use the strength of both arms to rotate the shoulders further in the stretch direction.

For an additional strengthening effect, the exercise can be done in the standing, crouched position. Lower yourself to the approximate height the hips would be if you were sitting, and follow the same directions.

Photograph 2 shows a variation of the exercise as described. The basic rotation movement may be refined by how you position the body in relation to the knees. The second photograph shows me stretching in the opposite direction, but with my body much closer to one leg than the other. This additional angle moves the maximum stretch to above the hip you are stretching away from. Experiment with your own variations; you will find a variety of pleasing stretches within this simple format.

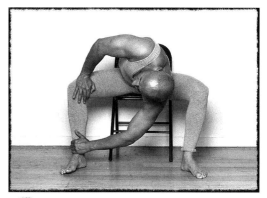

1 Body in between legs

Notes

hold ankle; brace against other leg

use arm strength to rotate shoulders

keep body in between knees

C–R: while holding, try to twist out of the position

use arms to restretch after breath out

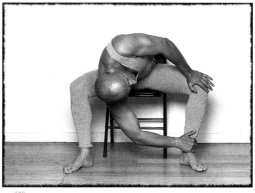

2 Variation with body closer to leg

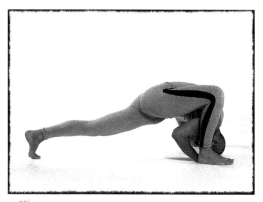

1 Final position of exercise 5

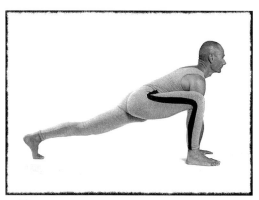

2 Advanced

Notes

keep hips level with floor

pull back on hands to straighten back

lower hips as far as you can

C–R: press front foot into floor

breathe in; relax, breathe out, and

let arms bend, take head towards floor

25. *Advanced buttock and hip flexors*

Take a moment to review exercise 5. The **advanced** version of the movement increases the stretch in the front leg's hip, and stretches the muscles of the lower back as well.

You are in the final position of exercise 5. Pull back on the hands while lifting the chest and looking to the front: these actions straighten the back, and will increase the sensations in both the front of the back leg, and the back of the front leg. Pause for a moment, and keeping the hips level and the back leg straight, let your hips go as low to the floor as you can.

A **C–R stretch** can improve movement at the front leg's hip. In the stretch position, try to press the front foot *into the floor* gently. This action engages all the muscles illustrated in exercise 5. Hold the contraction for five seconds and restretch, while keeping the hips level to avoid the tendency for the hip of the straight leg to sink to the floor.

Take a breath in, and as you breathe out let the arms bend further, and this time also let the head go forward until the lower back is stretched too. Advanced students will be able to put their foreheads on the floor with the back leg straight and the hips level. Hold the final position for a few full breaths in and out. This position is strenuous, and the supporting arms will be working hard. To come out of the position, always take a breath in and hold it in until you stand up. This will reduce the tendency to feel lightheaded—always a possibility when doing a difficult movement with the head lower than the heart. Rest for a moment or two before stretching the other side.

26. External hip rotator (piriformis)

To warm up for this **advanced** movement, practice exercise 9, and your choice from the *piriformis* exercises (6, 7 & 8), because this exercise requires suppleness in both the hip flexors (*iliacus* and *psoas*) and the external hip rotators. An explanation of the involvement of *piriformis* in sciatica and back pain can be found in chapter one, *Diagnosing your problem*. *piriformis* is one of the external hip rotators, small muscles deep in the hip near the joint, and which we use to turn the leg outwards.

A partner can make this movement extremely effective, by holding the hip of the front leg on the floor and leaning weight on the hip of the back leg. The partner has to help you to try to get your hips level; accordingly, their weight must be used on, or below, the hip joint, and their effort needs to be applied *across and down*. Even if you are strong, it is very difficult to apply leverage to your own body in this position to move the back leg's hip across, and doing this is essential for success in the exercise. The effort needed to hold yourself in the stretch position is similarly reduced with a partner's help.

The exercise is described for the hip of the left leg. Sit as shown. Your upper body's weight will be supported by your left hand. The objective of the movement is to roll the front of the right leg *across and forwards* while keeping the left hip on the floor, with the thighs parallel as might be seen from above. The effect of this movement is to provide a strong stretch deep inside the left hip, and a strong stretch in the right hip flexors in some people. The knee angle should be 90 degrees.

If you feel discomfort in the knee in the process of getting the hips level, you should use exercises 6 and 7 until the external hip rotators are sufficiently flexible to reduce the twisting effort on the knee. The force arises because we are using the lower leg to rotate the hip. Keep the trunk vertical as you get into the first position.

A **C–R stretch** can be used to improve the first position. Gently press the outside of the front foot into the floor for five seconds or so. This action contracts *piriformis*. Stop pressing, take a breath in, and on a breath out roll the right hip further across and down to the floor.

The second position requires the upper body to be bent

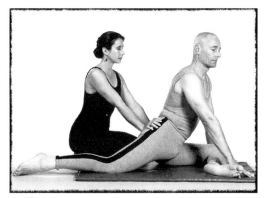

1   Partner presses hip *across and down*

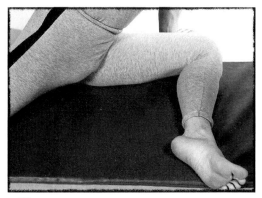

2   Knee angle is 90 degrees

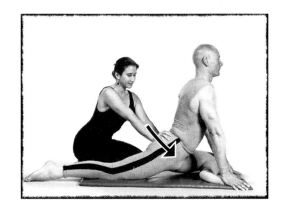

Notes

try to get hips level

C–R: press outside of foot into floor

try to get hips closer to level

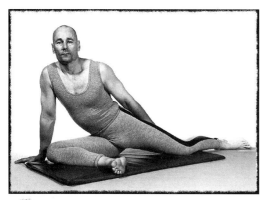

2 C–R: press outside of foot into floor

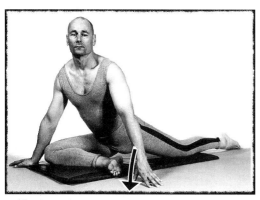

3 Lean over *ankle*

Notes

C–R: press outside of foot
into floor

after holding, lean forwards
over *ankle*

hold final position
for five breaths

forwards from the hip from the final stretch position you were able to achieve so far. You will notice that this movement is similar to the table-top hip exercise, number 8, but exercise 26 involves the hip flexors of the back leg. This is why this version is the strongest: the hip flexors being under intense stretch pull the top of the pelvis *forwards*, which moves the attachment point of *piriformis* away from its origin, thus increasing the stretch. Holding the back straight and the hips as level as possible, bend forwards from the hips, inclining the center of the body towards the *ankle* of the front foot, rather than towards the knee, the more comfortable direction. In fact, stretching over the knee reduces the stretch on *piriformis* significantly. Doing the exercise the recommended way will provide a powerful stretch for *piriformis* in the hip of the front leg, in addition to a stretch for the hip flexors of the back leg. For some people, the *adductors* (the muscles inside the front leg) will also be stretched. Change legs and compare the stretch sensations for each. Stretch whichever side is the more difficult a second time.

The **C–R stretch** may be performed again from the second position, by pressing the foot into the support surface. Stop pressing, relax, and after a breath in and out, incline the body further over the ankle. Hold for ten breaths and repeat for the other side.

27. Front thigh (quadriceps)

If the hip flexor exercise (the *iliopsoas* stretch, exercise 9 above) is difficult for you, you may include a stretch for *quadriceps* (the large muscles of the front of the thighs), as these muscles are likely to be tight too. One of the quadriceps, *rectus femoris,* is a hip flexor also, depending on leg position in relation to the body. Three quadriceps stretches are offered here, and any is a suitable warmup movement for the hip flexor stretch. I recommend strongly that a hip flexor stretch and a *quadriceps* stretch be practiced before doing any of the trunk backwards bending exercises.

Try the standing version first. This has a slightly different effect to the lying version that follows, as some extension of the leg is possible (with respect to the pelvis), and accordingly the top part of the thigh will be stretched in addition to the middle and lower sections. Stand opposite a wall as shown for balance, and lift the foot as close to the bottom as possible, and clasp the ankle. If you wish to stretch the instep as well, hold the toes. Bring the foot as close to the bottom as possible, and stand up straight. If you cannot hold the leg (due to tightness in the thigh), you can place the foot on a suitable support behind you, and stretch the thigh by shuffling back towards the support.

A partner can assist in the standing version, by placing one hand on the foot next to the bottom (pressing the foot closer), clasping the other hand around the knee of the bent leg, and gently pulling the knee back. The pulling movement should have the first hand as its pivot; that is, the first hand fixes the position of the foot and holds the hip forward, and the other pulls the thigh into the extension position. Two different **C–R stretches** are possible. The first is an attempt to straighten the held leg (for the usual five to ten seconds). The second is trying to pull the folded leg *forwards* away from the partner (towards the wall) for the same duration. The partner enhances the stretch by pressing the foot closer to your bottom, or by pulling the folded leg further in extension, or both. These C–R stretches may be done separately if the resulting stretch is too strong. Repeat for the other leg.

Jennifer is demonstrating a third version of the *quadriceps* stretch. Because you can control the degree of knee flexion by how close you take the hips to the wall, this version will be more comfortable in the knees for some people than the versions shown overleaf. Place a cushion or mat under the supporting knee. Ease the calf muscle of the leg against the wall out of the way (as shown overleaf), and move the hips backwards to feel the stretch. If you have a tendency to hyperextend in the lower back (very likely if *iliopsoas* are tight), press both hands down on the knee of the front leg as shown, and *tighten the abdominal muscles.* This action pulls the front of the pelvis upwards, flattens the lumbar spine and increases the

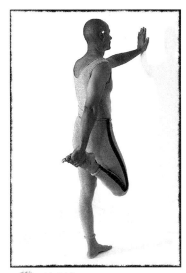

1 Hold foot

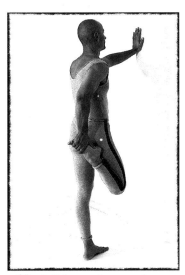

2 Pull foot to bottom, then

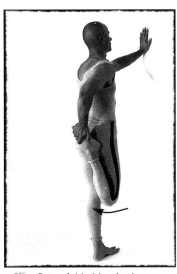

3 Bring folded leg *back*

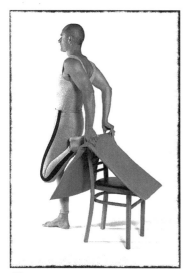

Alternative version

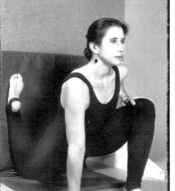

1 Easier on the knees than lying version overleaf

Notes

foot against wall

keep trunk straight

bring hips back to foot

tighten stomach muscles

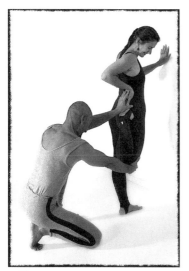

1 Partner version

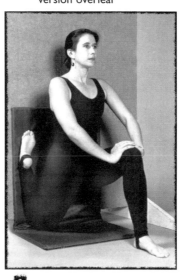

2

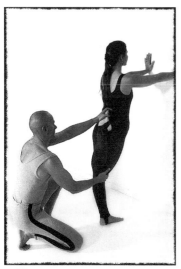

2

Notes

don't let your back
bend backwards

tighten stomach muscles

try to pull heel to buttock

stretch in the thigh muscle. Hold the body vertical and bring the body closer to the wall to increase the stretch.

The seated version of the thigh stretch has the advantage of being easier to hold for more extended periods. Look at photograph 1. When getting into this position, always push the calf muscle out of the way before bringing the foot close to the leg. (Both the calf and hamstring muscles, if tight, resist flowing out of the way in this position, and if this is the case the bulk of the muscles tends to force the knee joint apart. This tendency is exacerbated by exercising in pants that are too tight, or that do not stretch.) You must be able to sit with this buttock on the ground. If you cannot, place a firm cushion under the hip of the straight leg so that the hips remain level. The thicker the support, the less the stretch in the thigh. There should be no discomfort in the knee of the folded leg. The knees should stay close together, and the foot of the folded leg should point directly backwards.

Assuming that the position attained so far is comfortable, lean back onto the hands, then the elbows, to increase the stretch. Under no circumstances must you let the lower back hyperextend—if in doubt, tense the abdominal muscles and curl the body forwards. (Recall the remarks made about the iliopsoas muscles. These are stretched in this position, and if tight will pull the lumbar spine forward and hyperextend the back, which can be painful.)

To help stabilize the final position, and to help tilt the body's weight in the direction of the hip of the bent leg, you may bend the other leg and place the foot flat on the floor near the bottom, and grasp its ankle to hold it there. Refer to the accompanying photographs. This action makes holding the final position more comfortable and increases the stretch because the hips are held level. Lying in this way makes it more difficult to avoid the stretch in the folded leg, and the form is better preserved. This assistance technique may be used in the intermediate positions too, for increased effect. Hold the final position for at least ten normally paced breaths in and out.

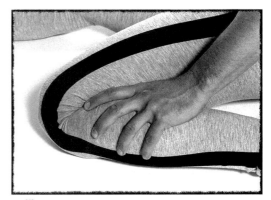

1 Push calf muscle out of the way

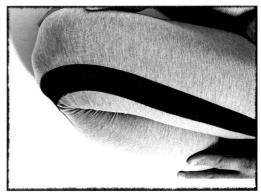

2 Bring hip across inside ankle

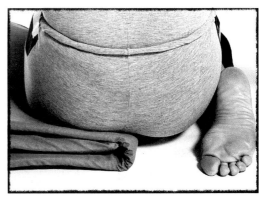

If you cannot sit with both buttocks on the ground

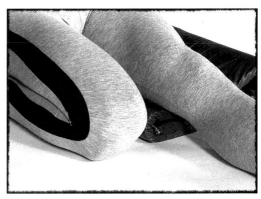

Above position, from front

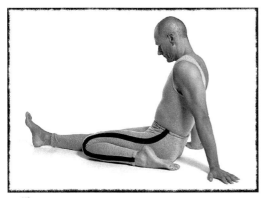

1

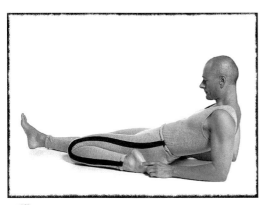

2

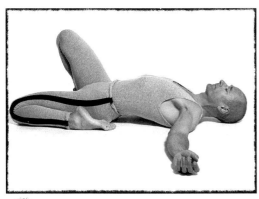

3 Do not let back arch backwards

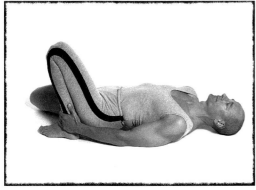

4 Hold ankle to keep hips level

Muscles of the front and inside of the leg

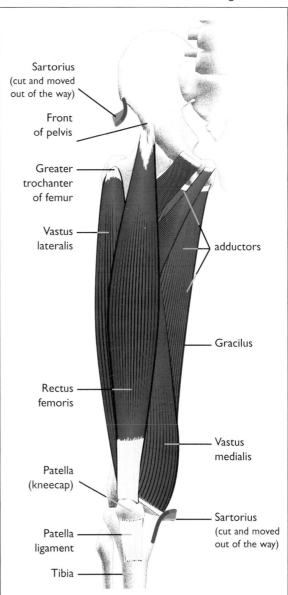

Sartorius
(cut and moved
out of the way)

Front
of pelvis

Greater
trochanter
of femur

Vastus
lateralis

adductors

Rectus
femoris

Gracilus

Vastus
medialis

Patella
(kneecap)

Sartorius
(cut and moved
out of the way)

Patella
ligament

Tibia

Notes

tighten stomach muscles
as you lean back

keep hips level

breathe normally

roll *away* from the stretch
to sit up

28. Backward bend over support

The recommendation to undertake backward bending exercises—often made to people suffering back pain—is not wise, as the great majority of back pain sufferers find these movements painful. Thus the forward bending and rotation exercises covered to this point should be used to relieve pain initially. However, to return one's back to full function, extension movements are also required. Such exercises should be included in your routine only when the original pain has subsided to the point where your daily movements are comfortable and relatively pain free. Use your discretion—and if the inclusion of extension movements irritates the recovering back structures, discontinue them until the discomfort reduces, and cautiously begin adding them again.

The advantages of the first suggested extension position are that because it requires no strength for its support it can be held for a considerable length of time (letting you relax into the stretch), and because the body is prone and supported along its length, there is minimal compression on the vertebrae.

You will need a firm support of suitable diameter, which will depend on one's length of trunk and flexibility. I am using an oil drum cut lengthways and padded, but any firm round surface may be used. For example, a cylindrical firm pillow of suitable diameter, or a small cushion on top of a larger firm cushion of sizes that will support about half the length of your back is satisfactory, but a firm support is preferable for your first attempts at backward bending.

Sit on the floor with your knees bent and your back to the support. Use your arms to lower yourself over the support until you are lying across it. After the body is supported along its length, let the neck extend fully, back onto an additional support if necessary. This precaution will prevent the neck from being overextended. Rest in this position for a few breaths and, when comfortable and relaxed, slowly raise the arms backwards until they are stretched out overhead. This is the final position. Hold it for ten breaths or so.

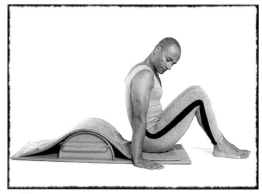

1

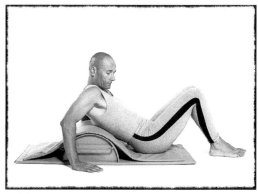

2 *Shoulders* over barrel midline

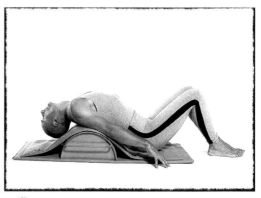

3

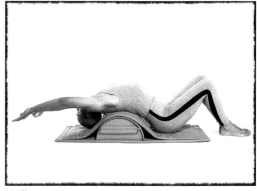

4 Reach arms out to increase stretch

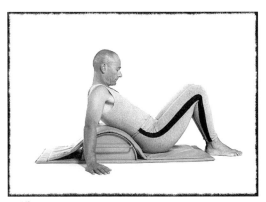

1 *Middle* back over barrel midline

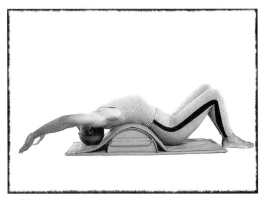

2 Reach arms out fully

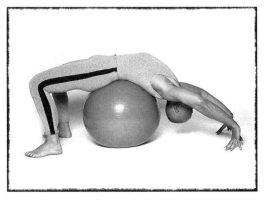

Legs apart for stability

Notes

try different start positions

relax into the position

C–R: gently initiate sitting-up movement

restretch after a breath out

roll to the *side* to get off the support

An optional **C–R stretch** may help relax the stomach muscles: from the stretch position, lift the head and initiate the sitting-up movement by lightly tensing the muscles involved for a few seconds (but do not lift the body from the support). Restretch, and hold the final position for at least ten breaths, relaxing completely.

To return to the start position, bring the arms back to your side, place them on the floor, and use them to lift yourself up into the sitting position. While doing this, try to keep the rest of the body relaxed—in particular, do not use the groin or stomach muscles to return yourself to the sitting position. This direction is to avoid using the hip flexors to sit up—doing so from this position may make the lower back feel very uncomfortable. An alternative method of sitting up is to roll slowly to the side before getting up. Experiment with your position on the support. The second sequence shows a body placement that emphasizes the middle and lower back, by placing the body further over the support to begin.

The last photograph shows a similar exercise, but done over an exercise ball. I have placed myself far enough over the ball to emphasize the stretch in the abdominal area; accordingly the lower back is most strongly extended. Have your feet well apart for stability. I will elaborate on the use of these balls below in exercises 35 and 36.

Assuming the exercise does not make the back feel worse, you may make the stretch stronger by using a higher support, or by slowly extending one leg at a time. When both legs are extended, breathe deeply and try to let the body relax completely.

When relaxed, you should feel the stretch in the abdominal area (the front of the body between the ribs and the hips), between the ribs and in the chest, too, when you raise the hands overhead. Regular practice of these kinds of movements will also help reduce the tendency for the upper back to bend forward and the shoulders hunch forward as you get older. These relatively passive extension movements prepare the body for the more difficult backwards bending movements. Exercise 1 or 14 may be used to relax back muscles that may have tightened doing the practice.

See exercise 33 for an additional upper and middle back extension movement.

29. Backward bend from floor

The next exercise is described in two forms, because one's proportion (lengths of body segments) substantially influences the final effects of the pose. The critical aspect of this pose is in keeping the lower back muscles completely relaxed while using only the arms to lift the shoulders and incline the upper body backwards.

This exercise, in various forms, has been a popular recommendation of physiotherapists. The underlying rationale is that if intervertebral disc material is bulging posteriorly, bending the spine backwards will "push" or "squeeze" the material back into place (through pressure from the bony structures of the vertebrae as they slide backwards over one another). The problem with this approach is that backward-bending movements commonly irritate the back pain sufferer, probably through compression of the same joints. Such compression sensations will be exacerbated by any tension in the muscles running along the spine. For this reason, exercises which relax these muscles should be used to reduce discomfort and improve mobility in the first instance, and backward-bending movements be added only when they can be performed reasonably comfortably. In time, when one becomes flexible in the lumbar spine bending backwards, the stretch will be felt in the abdominal muscles.

The conventional way to approach this stretch (the cobra pose in Yoga) is to tense the buttock muscles before starting and to hold these muscles tight during the pose. The problem with this direction is that the untrained person cannot avoid tensing the lower back muscles as well—the very thing we are trying to avoid.

The **easiest version:** the starting position is lying face-down, legs together, with your hands flat on the floor underneath the shoulders. Deliberately relax the whole body. Take a deep breath in, and as you begin to breathe out, use only the arm muscles to elevate the upper body slowly onto one elbow at a time, leaving the front of the hips on the floor. Use your partner to monitor any tightening of the lower back muscles, by asking them to place a hand on these muscles just above the bottom. As soon as any significant tightening is detected, lower yourself a fraction, relax, and try again. Rest on the elbows with the head in a neutral position with respect to the trunk, and let the front of the

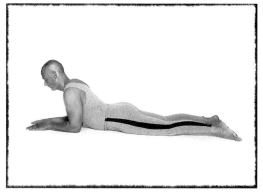

Easiest

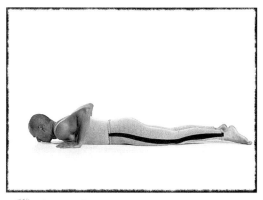

1 Intermediate

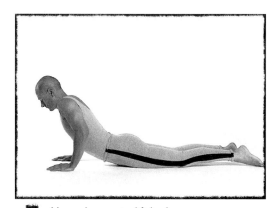

2 Use only *arms* to lift body

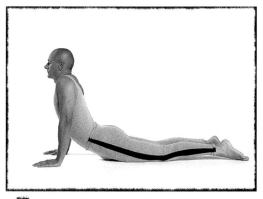

3 Open mouth before tilting head back

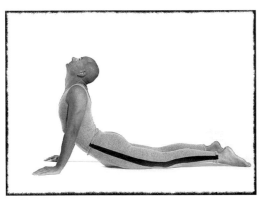

4   Final position (includes a neck stretch)

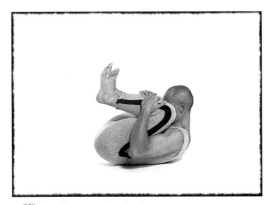

5   Roll up to relax back

Notes

keep all back muscles soft

begin again if muscles
tighten up

pull shoulders back
to tighten position

head back to finish

try to breathe normally

body sink as close as it can to the floor. Breathe ten slow breaths.

In the **intermediate version,** start the same way, but extend the arms. If you think that you may not be flexible enough to extend the arms fully, place your hands further out to the *sides,* so that your shoulders will not be lifted quite as high when the arms are straightened. If you can keep the lower back muscles relaxed, this is an effective and comfortable stretch for the front of the body. As soon as you have reached maximum arm extension, pause and breathe in and out a few times, trying to keep the body as relaxed as possible. Breathe in, and draw the shoulders as far back as you can, using the muscles of the shoulder blades and upper back. Be careful that this action does not tense the muscles of the lower back. If it does, lower yourself to the floor and begin again, concentrating on the first part of the exercise only. Hold the final position for ten breaths.

Once comfortable in the final position, the stretch may be enhanced by opening the mouth and tilting the head back. Once the head is back, slowly close the mouth. Hold this position for a few breaths in and out.

The recovery position is shown in the final photograph. Always finish backward bending by coming out of it *slowly* and immediately rolling over onto your back and clasping the bent knees to the chest. This action will gently stretch the lower back muscles, which usually (despite one's best efforts) will have tightened up a little during the pose. Hold the knees to the chest until the lower back feels relaxed. Any of the forward bending or rotation exercises (1, 2, 3, 13 or 14) can be substituted for the knees to the chest movement if you prefer.

A variation is referred to as the "suspended" version. Begin in the push-up position—the body's weight supported on straight arms and on the balls of the feet, with the body held straight. Look at the photographs. Lower yourself into the stretch position by letting the body relax and by letting the body's weight bring the hips towards the floor. The only parts of the body exerting any force should be the muscles at the back of the arms, used to keep the arms straight. On no account should the back muscles be tight—rather, slowly let them go completely slack and let gravity bring the hips to the floor, taking your time. Notice that the body sinks between the shoulders too (this requires that the muscles of the trunk, including the muscles under the arms, be relaxed). As soon as the thighs touch the floor, carefully straighten the legs so that you are suspended between hands and feet. The head should be in the neutral position at this point. Providing the lower back feels comfortable, cautiously bring the shoulders back. This instruction is given because pulling the shoulders back tends to tighten the lower back muscles, which we do not want. If this happens, redo the pose without this last action. Rest in the final position of the movement for at least five breaths in and out.

Notes

lower body slowly

when hips touch floor, straighten legs

suspend body between hands and feet

pull shoulders back

take head back to finish

roll up to relax back

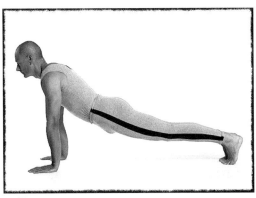

1

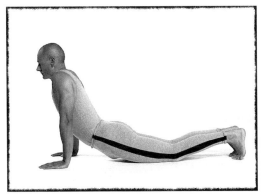

2 Straighten legs to gain elevation

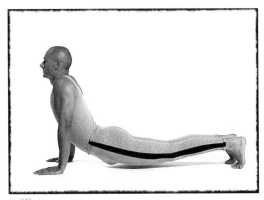

3 Lean back to increase stretch

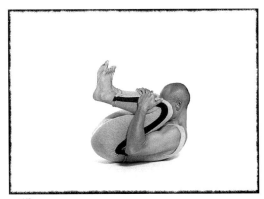

4 Roll up to relax back

30. Standing calf

In addition to the conventional forward bending movements, another exercise with beneficial effects on the sciatic nerve is one that specifically stretches the calf muscles. If sciatica is a problem, you should include this exercise in your routine. Whereas the hamstring stretch (exercise 11) derived its effect on the sciatic nerve from flexion of both the hip and ankle joints, this exercise concentrates on the ankle.

Place yourself facing a wall as shown. The front foot is used for stability only. Support yourself on outstretched hands while bent forward at the hips with the back held straight. Place the back foot three feet or more away from the wall. If supporting yourself on your arms is too tiring, you can rest on the elbows and forearms instead with no loss of effect on the ankle. Press the back leg straight (necessary to stretch the top calf muscle, *gastrocnemius*). While holding the heel firmly on the floor, move the hips towards the wall until you feel sufficient stretch. Each calf muscle supports at least our whole body's weight daily, and is often resistant to being stretched, so hold the final stretch for a minimum of a ten-breath cycle.

It is essential that the foot of the leg being stretched is directly *in front of* the shin. It is a common mistake in this exercise to either place the foot slightly at an angle out to the side, or to permit the ankle to roll inwards (*pronate*). Letting the ankle roll in this way avoids the proper stretch, and places an asymmetrical stretching force on the Achilles tendon, which (potentially) could be dangerous. If you have a tendency to do this, press a little extra weight onto the outside (little toe side) of the foot, and keep an eye on the shape of the ankle.

A **C–R stretch** can be very effective in loosening tight calf muscles. Once in the stretch position, gently press the ball of the foot into the floor for five seconds or so, but still keep the heel on the floor—an isometric contraction for the calf muscles, in other words. Relax, breathe in, and on a breath out, press the heel to the floor and take the hips a little closer to the wall. This is a strong stretch. Hold the final position for at least ten breaths.

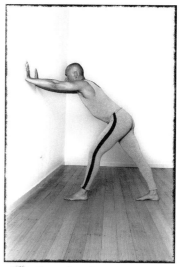

1 Front foot for stability only

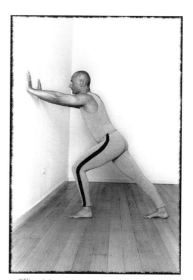

2 Move hips towards the wall

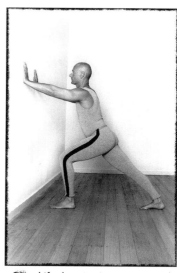

3 Lift chest to increase stretch

Notes

press back leg straight

back foot pointing
straight ahead

don't let ankle roll in

C–R: press toes of back
foot into floor

restretch after breath out

hold final position
for 30 seconds minimum

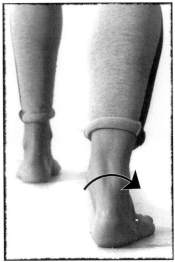

Avoid processes by pressing down
on little toe side

Sciatic nerve runs down
back of leg

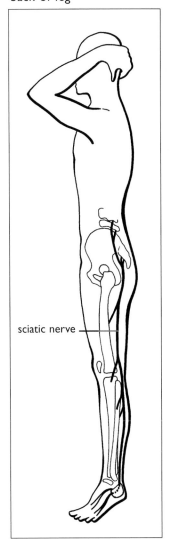

sciatic nerve

Muscles of the lower leg

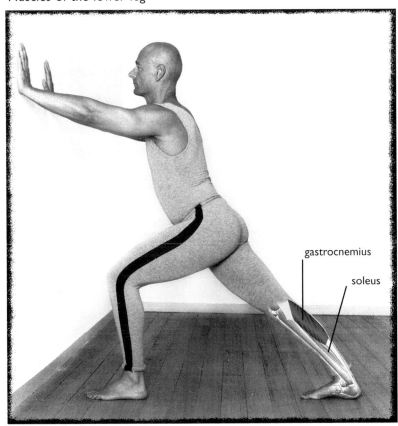

gastrocnemius

soleus

31. *Standing side bend*

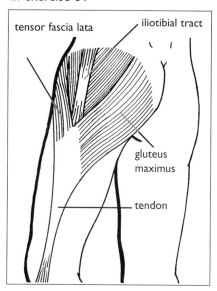

tensor fascia lata   iliotibial tract

gluteus maximus

tendon

Using a wall in this movement ensures correct alignment and provides support. The aim is to stretch all of the side waist muscles, the *obliques*, in the first instance. As these become more flexible, the exercise will also stretch one half of the *quadratus lumborum* pair and half of the deep spinal muscles, which may be involved in back pain. The abductors of the leg will also be stretched, including *tensor fascia lata*.

Standing with the weight evenly on both feet, lean the body against the wall. Use a chair off to one side to lean on if you feel vulnerable in the movement. Maintain the whole body in contact with the wall during the exercise. Lean to one side as far as you can, and grasp the leg. Two hand positions are shown—choose the one that gives you the best support. Leaning on this hand, reach the other arm out and over the head as far as you can—the locus of the stretch will extend from above the hip you are stretching to the whole of that side. Hold the final position for five breaths only.

To come out of the stretch, very slowly *roll the top shoulder away from the wall*, trying to increase the sidewards stretch all the while. As you rotate the shoulder forward, your apparent flexibility at the waist will increase noticeably, and you will need to increase the lean to the side just to maintain the stretch sensation. The locus of the stretch will move too, from just above the hip to further towards the spine itself as the shoulder rotates forward. If you find a position that feels particularly good in this transition, pause there for a breath or two. Repeat for the other side.

The second sequence is an effective variation, if you have a support you can hang from. Stand with your feet under the shoulder closest to the support, and let the body hang from the arm. To increase the stretch, take the top arm towards the support as far as you can. Hold this position for a few breaths. To move the stretch from the side of the waist to the spine, let the inside hip roll back *very slowly*, maintaining the lean intensity. If you lean forwards slightly at the same time, a pleasing stretch of two small hip muscles (*gluteus minimus* and *medius*) and down to over the *sacro-iliac joint* can be achieved. Hold the final position for five breaths, and pull yourself back to the start position with the support arm. A muscle to the front of the hip, *tensor fascia lata*, may be stretched by rolling the inside hip *forwards* slightly from the starting position. This can be an effective stretch for people with *iliotibial band* problems. **C–R stretches** may be effected by pressing the outside foot *away* from you into the floor, and leaning further into the stretch direction.

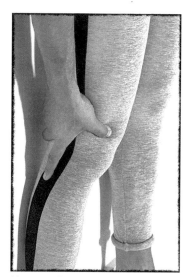

You must be able to *lean* on the support hand

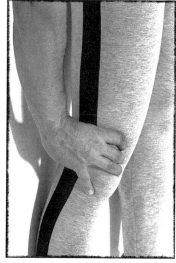

Alternative grip, better for thicker legs

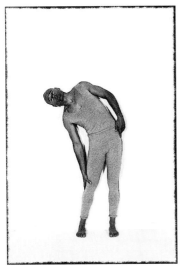

1 Lean onto hand

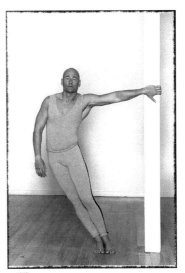

1

Notes (left)

grasp leg and *lean* on support hand

stretch top arm out

roll shoulder forward to return

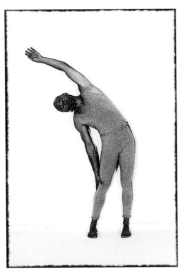

2 Full stretch to the side

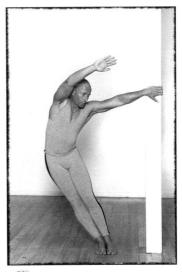

2 Rotate hips to move stretch

Notes (right)

hang all your weight from arm

let hips stretch away from support

hold initial stretch for a few breaths

let inside hip roll *backwards* or *forwards* to move stretch

pull yourself out of the stretch with holding arm

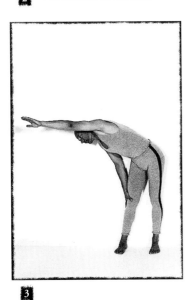

3

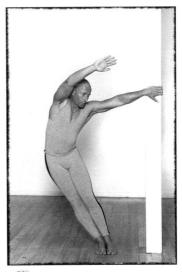

3

32. Lying side bend

The previous stretch may be too strong if your back is sensitive. Bending to the side while standing requires the facet joints of the lumbar spine to slide over each other and, under compression, pain may result. Exercise 32 removes much of this load, but requires careful positioning and some strength in the arms for support. The main effect of this exercise is on the hip abductors. This exercise may be useful for those who are tight in this area—broadly speaking, from the lower back to mid-thigh, as occurs frequently in runners. A wall may also be used to maintain alignment in this version.

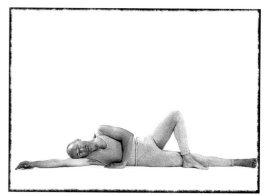

1

There are two ways of getting into the position shown. The first (requiring more arm strength but permitting more control) is to lie on the floor on one side with hips, legs, and shoulders in line. You may use a wall for alignment the first time you practice the movement to get used to its dynamics, but if you do, you will not be able to move the hips easily if you want to move the stretch. Place the hands as shown, and achieve the required stretch by pushing the hands away from the body, raising the body without letting the hip leave the floor. The arm of the shoulder furthest from the hips will do most of the work. If comfortable, you may use the waist muscles of the side you are bending towards to assist the lifting movement. The top leg may be bent and placed in front of the other for stability. If you use the top waist muscles for assistance, be sure to relax the muscles, by repeating the stretch briefly on the side you begin with after doing the second side. Roll the top hip forwards and backwards a little to find the most effective stretch.

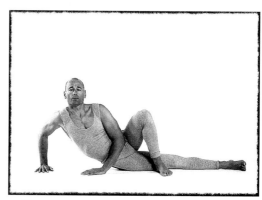

2 Lift body by arms only

The second way begins by resting on the outstretched arm with the body held straight, as shown. The foot of the top leg is used for support, by placing it in front of you. Slowly let the body bend at the waist until you feel the required stretch. Rest in this position for five breaths or so. Repeat for the other side. The stretch may be moved by rolling the top leg's hip forwards or backwards slightly.

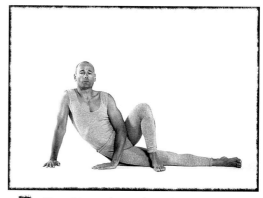

3 Move hip to change desired stretch

C–R stretches may be done in both versions, by pressing the outside of the straight leg's foot directly down into the floor for five seconds or so, and restretching.

If you do not get sufficient stretch from either of these approaches (it may be, for example, that you have relatively short arms and a long trunk), you may intensify the effect

Notes

hand directly under shoulder

lift slowly

lean *away* from support hand to increase stretch

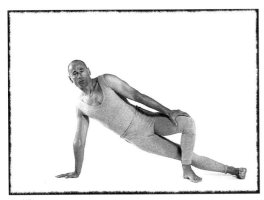

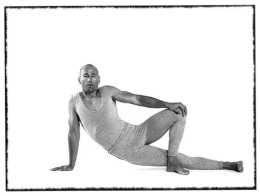

1

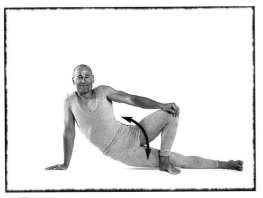

2 Lower body by waist muscles

3 Hip forwards or backwards to move stretch

Notes

lower yourself *slowly*

use foot to move hips
to move stretch

breathe normally

by resting your supporting hand on a block or similar object. Alternatively, the supporting foot may be rested on the block. Using a block under the hand tends to concentrate the stretch above the waist. Conversely, a block under the foot tends to move the point of maximum stretch below the hip joint. Experiment and choose the one that works best for you.

As both versions are shown (with the top hip directly over the bottom hip), the stretch will be felt on the outside of, and above, the bottom hip. To move the stretch forwards, roll the top hip forwards by walking the foot of the bent leg forwards; similarly, to move the stretch on the bottom hip backwards, roll the top hip backwards. In this way, the exercise can stretch a great number of hip and lower back muscles. Make these movements small, as even tiny movements can change which muscles will be affected.

33. Middle and upper back backward bend

Slumping of the shoulders and rounding of the upper back are common postural problems. Both these changes are extremely common phenomena accompanying aging. A reduction in the suppleness of the muscles between the ribs (*intercostals*) and a shortening of the front arm muscles (*biceps brachii*), the front shoulder muscles (*anterior deltoids*), and the chest muscles (*pectoralis major* and *minor*) are significant factors in these changes.

The role of these changes in neck pain is easy to imagine, and is seen everywhere. Any increased forward bending of the upper back results either in an increase in the backwards curvature of the cervical spine (and possible increased compression of the facet joints) or the carrying of the head forward of its normal balanced position (requiring the posterior neck muscles to do more work to maintain posture in any position). Such extra effort means that these muscles reach their work limit before they otherwise would. Here, work limit may be as simple as getting tired, or feeling noticeable tension.

Notes

relax into the stretch position

press arms up away from you

C–R: try to press your hands *into* the wall

breathe normally in the stretch position

Upper body muscles

Changes accompanying aging

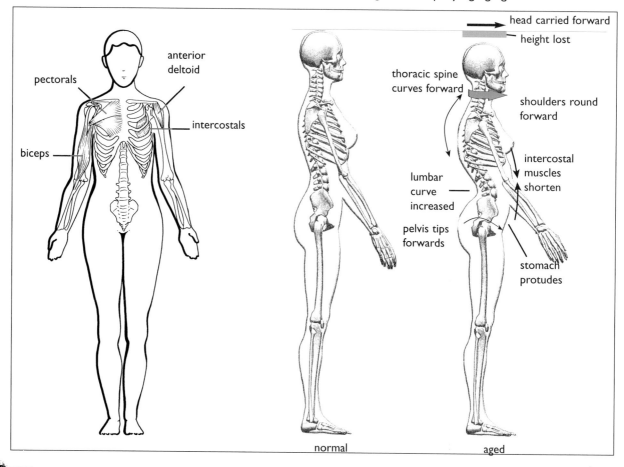

normal

aged

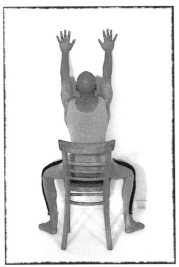

2 C–R direction

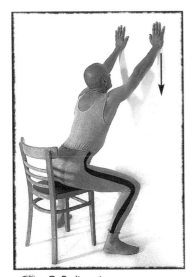

3 Partner may apply a light force here

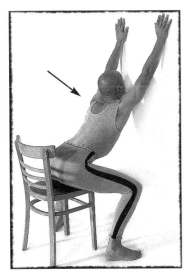

1 Shoulder-width hand spacing

The role such changes may have in low back pain is less obvious. It is probably related to load redistribution necessitated by changes to the shape of the spine, and the additional strain placed on the lumbar vertebrae if the function of any other part of the spine is reduced. Whenever the head is carried forward of the center of gravity, the muscles of the back are required to do additional work. On the workshops we have noticed that people with increased curvature of the thoracic spine frequently demonstrate tight hip flexors. Whether the curvature is the result of tightening of the hip flexors and tilting of the pelvis, or whether the state of the hip flexors is the result of the increased curvature is an open question.

The purpose of the following poses (including the stronger partner C–R versions) is to "open" the chest and increase the capacity of the middle and upper back to bend backwards. Open, used in this way, means to counter the normal (though undesirable) shortening of the muscles mentioned. After a period of practice, the shoulders will sit further back on the rib cage without conscious effort and the chest will appear and feel expanded.

The **easiest** version uses a chair and a wall, and may be done in the office if you wish. Look at the photographs. As the body's weight is supported by the chair, this version is less strenuous than the following exercises. Place the chair at a distance from the wall which gives you the intensity of stretch you require. Look at a spot in between your hands. This will help initiate a bend backwards in the upper back by involving the *trapezius* muscles in the upper back. Here too, a partner can make the stretch more intense if desired, by placing his or her hand on the most forward-curved part of the middle or upper back and applying a little weight.

A **C–R stretch** can be achieved by gently trying to *pull* the hands down the wall against friction, once in the stretch position. To restretch, take a breath in, relax completely, and on a breath out let your body's weight do the work.

The **intermediate** version requires only something to kneel on, if you are working on a hard floor—a folded blanket is ideal. Kneel and walk yourself forward on your hands until the arms are fully extended in front of you at about shoulder width. Note that some people will need a slightly wider or narrower hand position to take the strain off the shoulders. Press the arms straight, extending them from the body as far as you can. Move forward on your hands until the hips are *directly over* the knees. Relax the legs. Look at the floor between your hands, take a deep breath, and on an exhalation let the upper body sink as close to the floor as it can. Keep the arms extended—the tendency will be to let the elbows bend and that will dissipate the effects of the pose. This is quite a subtle position and you will not derive the benefits until you let the body's own weight bring you closer to the floor. Hold the final position for ten to fifteen breaths in and out. To return to the starting position, bring your hands back to under the shoulders, come up to a hands and knees position, and fold the body over the legs. Rest in this final position for a few breaths.

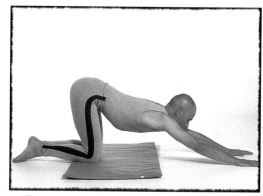

1

Even solo, a **C–R stretch** can yield surprising improvements in the final stretch position. The contraction that you use here will be extremely gentle, though; recall that one of the two principles that must be observed is that when contracting, the body must not move at all. In this solo version of the C–R stretch the body will be lifted if you press too hard, so press with just enough force to *feel* the muscles involved. These will be the muscles under the arm (*latissimus dorsi*) primarily, with the abdominal, rib and chest muscles secondarily. After contracting, take a deep breath in, and as you breathe out relax completely, and let gravity take your chest to the floor.

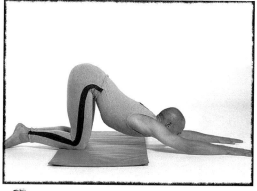

2

The next most intense **intermediate** version is the floor movement with a partner. Consider the photographs opposite. The partner is kneeling between my outstretched hands, with both hands placed on my upper back between my shoulder blades. The partner, as always, must be in a position that guarantees stable weight and permits quick removal of the applied weight if necessary. For this reason, the partner has her right foot forwards for stability. The partner does not press her weight, but rather is *leaning* her weight on me. Notice that her arms are placed at about 90 degrees from the part of my back she is leaning on. Because of the shape of my back, this angle results in about half of

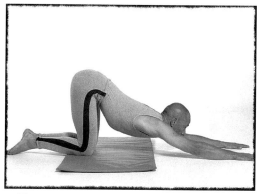

3

Notes

extend arms as far as possible

look between hands

relax to let body sink to floor

C–R: press hands into floor

relax and breathe

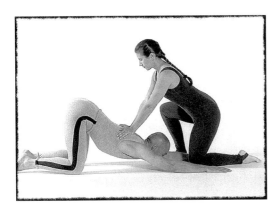

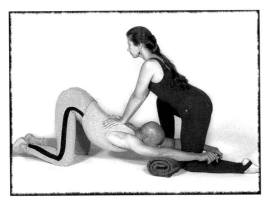

Elbows on support for clearance

Notes

supply weight to roundest
part of back

C–R: press hands into floor

relax and breathe out

partner gently applies
more weight

her weight pressing down to the floor (extending the arms with respect to the body) and about half pressing back to my hips (helping the back to bend backwards).

Relax completely while keeping the arms pressed straight so that the upper body is pressed towards the floor. Hold the final position for five breaths. When being stretched in this position, it is essential that the partner does not lean too much weight on you. If you are tensing up against the weight it is probably too much.

A **C–R stretch** will provide a stronger effect if required. Once in the final stretch position you may gently press your hands down onto the floor for about five seconds, using the whole body. This contracts all the muscles described in the first paragraph, and that we are trying to stretch. With an exhalation, relax completely. You may need to ask your partner to lean a little more weight on you in the relaxed position to feel sufficient stretch. Hold the final position for five breaths in and out. The last photograph shows a variation which may be used if the chest contacts the floor before the desired stretch is experienced. The elbows are placed on a rolled-up mat or similar object. This version can be more comfortable in the shoulders for some people. Try all versions, and select the one that gives the best effects.

The **advanced** standing version seems to stretch the muscles under the arms more than the floor version. Even done solo it is a much stronger stretch than the versions above as more of the body's weight is experienced on the hands. The disadvantage is some people will experience an uncomfortable compression sensation in the lumbar spine. If this happens, move your feet slightly closer to the wall, and try again. It is necessary to be able to relax the muscles on the front of the upper body, so you need to be relatively comfortable in the position.

Stand three feet or so away from a wall, facing it. Place the hands on the wall about eighteen inches or so above the shoulders. Bend the legs slightly to remove the hamstring stretching aspect and to remove compression from the lower back. Look up between your hands (this slightly tenses the *trapezius* muscles and helps to extend the upper back). Press the arms out and away from the body as though you are trying to reach through the wall (this stretches the muscles under the arms, *latissimus dorsi*, and the chest muscles). Lean into the wall so that the body's weight is felt on the shoulders, and the upper back bends backwards. Rest with the body's weight on the arms and breathe in and out deeply five times or so.

You may use a partner in this version too, in two ways. The first is to use a small amount of your partner's weight to increase the standard stretch. Placement of the partner's weight is determined by the shape of your back. In general, the partner should place his or her weight on the part of the middle or upper back that is the least flexible (that is, most rounded forwards). Have your partner use the flat of the forearm or the hands as shown to transfer the required weight, applying just enough weight to make the exercise strong enough for you. Using a partner tends to concentrate the effect at the point where the weight is applied, and permits you to relax fully in the position. Hold the final position for five breaths or so.

The **C–R standing version**, a very strong exercise indeed, uses the partner's weight as resistance against which to contract. Here, without letting them slide, try to pull the hands down the wall. This action will contract the muscles mentioned above. Hold for five seconds or so, and *cautiously and slowly* let yourself relax into the full stretch, ensuring that the arms are pressed completely straight. You must ask your partner to apply his or her weight very sensitively, as this is an extended position where the leverage factors strongly favor the partner. Experiment with different hand spacings too, to find the one most comfortable for the shoulders. Generally, the closer the hands, the stronger the stretch.

All versions of this exercise are backward-bending movements, and as such are likely to tighten muscles in the upper or lower back. Back muscles tend to tighten if work is demanded of them towards the contracted end of their range of movement, and most people find it

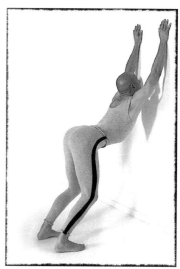
1 Lean into wall to stretch

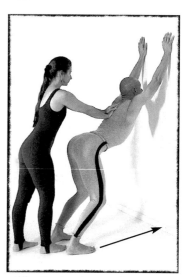
2 Further from wall

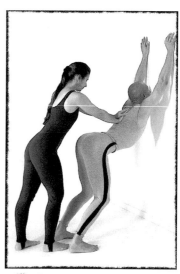
3 Partner assist

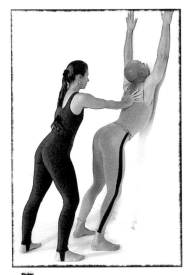

1

difficult to keep these muscles relaxed while doing movements of this kind. Accordingly, you will feel most comfortable if you follow these exercises with a forward-bending movement.

If the lower back tightens, use exercise 1, or the recovery position of exercise 29 to relax. If the upper back has tightened, do exercise 13 or 14 to relax the muscles involved.

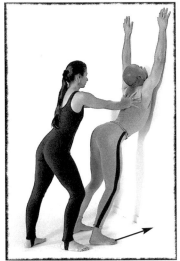

2 Try different spacing of feet from wall to find most comfortable position

Notes

supply small weight to roundest part of back

C-R: try to pull hands down wall

relax and breathe out

let body go towards wall

STRENGTHENING EXERCISES

This introduction provides a brief note about strength training, and a few suggestions about setting a goal for yourself. As noted in the previous chapters, knowing *why* one is doing something a certain way is just as important as knowing *how*. Details of numbers of repetitions of exercises and frequency of training are set out in the *Planning a total routine* section at the end of this chapter.

When one hears talk of strength training, it usually refers to *isotonic* exercise, which uses muscle effort against a resistance that can move. Such forces may be generated to push or pull a weight or some other kind of resistance (*concentric* contractions), or to resist the movement of some object (as in lowering something heavy to the floor, called *eccentric* contractions). Both approaches are effective in building strength. This method of strength training is not new. Milos of Croton, a famous wrestler of ancient Greece, was said to have lifted a bull calf overhead every day until it was fully grown. We do not necessarily need extensive gym equipment to do isotonic training. The body itself can be effective resistance, as in doing chin-ups or similar exercises. The design of the body lends itself to using its own weight for most of the trunk strengthening exercises that we will be considering below.

There is no doubt that isotonic training is successful, and this approach to strength training is the method of choice of the overwhelming majority of athletes who need strength for their sports. Nonetheless, even though there is positive visual and physical feedback to this kind of training, you will still require motivation. One needs to persevere with strength training for more than two months, which seems to be a critical point for many people. Many gym owners have mentioned to me that they make a good fraction of their income from those people who sign up for a year's membership in January, full of New Year's resolutions, and who are never seen after February. We have found that if a student perseveres with his or her routine for two months, the drop-out rate from the strength classes we teach is very small.

Matching training to expected demand

On a general note, there seems to be a threshold phenomenon in most people's approach to exercise—none or too much. My intention here is to mention a few common-sense suggestions upon which to base a training schedule to suit you. The main reasons exercise regimens fail are because there is no clearly visualized goal (purpose) to the program, or because the exercise program is inappropriate. By "inappropriate," I mean one that either is unrealistic in terms of how much time and energy will be needed on a weekly basis to do it, or one that is unsuited to your real needs. I will explore these ideas in more detail, following the last exercise in this chapter.

Without a goal, any exercise program is likely to become perfunctory at best, or mechanical and unfeeling at worst. Either disposition means little incentive to continue, and an increased risk of injury. Too often, people with the best and apparently the strongest of intentions cease their routines after a week or two. Those of you who have had a neck or back problem are usually more motivated to continue, at least while the exercises seem to be alleviating the problem. Unfortunately, ending the program when you get better is leaving the job half done. Your "pre-injury state of fitness" was precisely the set of physical characteristics that contributed to the problem in the first place. It is necessary to *strengthen* the body against the likelihood of a recurrence. If this is your goal, you do not need a comprehensive gym training program, but you do need a number of specific strengthening exercises of the sort that can be done at home. The critical point is that you do need to *do* them. And if you are successful in overcoming your original problem, and you feel drawn to explore the possibilities of self-improvement at your local gym, so much the better. The point is that you need to be clear in your own mind why you are doing what you do.

Low back pain is common among athletes. Certain sports are prone to this problem (sweep rowing, for example) due to the asymmetrical nature of the activity. Other athletes merely require strong waist muscles to transfer power or strength from one half of the body to the other. Athletes should explore the whole range of strengthening exercises presented. If you are a weekend athlete, such as a golf or tennis player, and you have a history of back or neck problems, you will need a few exercises in addition to the basic ones, and stronger movements will be found towards the end of this chapter. Activities like golf or tennis, with their demands on spinal extension with rotation, require strong waist and back muscles. The uneven strength requirements of these sports compound any tendency to back or neck problems, but if sufficient torso strength is developed, such activities can be pursued safely. The more effective (higher intensity) exercises will be required, and although the exercises are shown in a gymnasium setting, a little ingenuity will allow you to perform them at home, if you wish.

34. Abdominal curl

This is the basic abdominal strengthening exercise, and is often referred to as the "crunch." Some years ago, researchers in the United States realized that the conventional sit-up exercise (wherein one's feet were held under a support with either straight or bent knees and the body lifted up until the face contacted the knees) was potentially very harmful to the lower back. However, whenever you visit a gym, you will see this movement being done. You should appreciate why this exercise is both bad for the back and an inefficient abdominal strengthening exercise.

Any sitting-up movement (used as a strength exercise) where the lower back is lifted from the floor can place a strain on the lower back. The hip flexors play a role as shapers of the lumbar lordosis, and in the inability of some people to lie face-up with the lower back on the floor (see exercise 9). Anatomically (*psoas* and *iliacus* will be considered as one muscle for simplicity), the hip flexors originate in the transverse processes of the lumbar spine and insert at the top of the femur. This means that when they contract strongly against fixed legs (as in the conventional sit-up) the body's weight is lifted from the front of the lower back. This is a *class II lever*, with the effort between fulcrum and load, as shown in the illustration. The main significance of this class of lever, with respect to the arrangement of the bones of the spine, is the generation in the lumbar vertebrae of powerful *shear* forces, which can disturb their ideal position. Additionally, if the abdominal muscles are weak (the usual reason for doing the exercise) the upper body is apt to lag slightly behind the waist as the body is lifted, and this hyperextends the spine while compressing it. Compression forces alone can irritate the facet joints, whose articular surfaces are rich in nerves. In most people the hip flexors are far stronger than the abdominal muscles. If stabilizing the pelvis in the horizontal plane is one of our goals, this strength imbalance needs to be addressed. The conventional sit-up will only increase the imbalance, as its major effect is to strengthen the hip flexors. It is only when the abdominal muscles are really strong that this exercise can be done without the lower back taking the strain. In any case, this exercise should be avoided by anyone with back problems.

Consider the anatomy of the abdominal muscles for a moment (for simplicity only the *rectus abdominis* will be

Why the conventional situp can injure the lower back

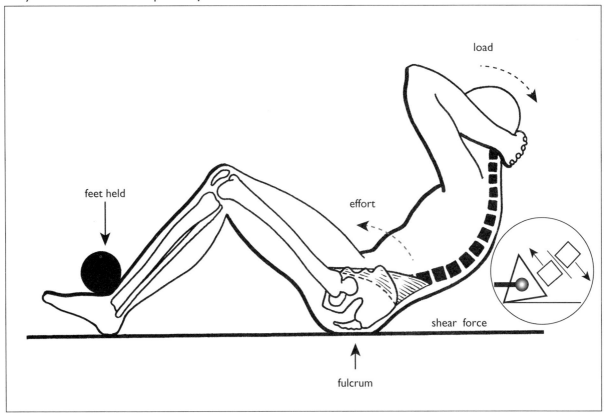

feet held

load

effort

shear force

fulcrum

Class II lever

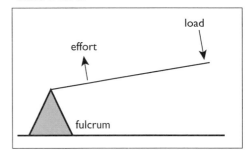

effort

load

fulcrum

mentioned). Their origin is the cartilage of the lower ribs; their insertion is the pubic bone. Their only action therefore is to bring the ribs closer to the pubic bone (or the pubic bone closer to the ribs if the ribs are fixed)—they have no direct role in hip flexion at all. To be effective as a strengthener of the abdominal muscles, the sit-up exercise needs to be redesigned. In the conventional sit-up, the only part of the movement that can strengthen these muscles is actually avoided. If the movement is done quickly (as it usually is when people are trying to do as many repetitions as possible), the action of lifting the head off the floor rapidly is initiated by the neck, arm and back muscles. This momentum is used to help the abdominal muscles contract as the shoulders are lifted from the floor, and the hip flexors take over to complete the movement.

The only way to make this an abdominal exercise is to isolate the abdominal muscles. This is done by flexing the hips as shown (the lower legs may be rested on a chair for greater comfort), and doing the exercise *slowly*. Place just the fingertips on the temples (this stops you lifting the head with your arms), and slowly lift the head up with the muscles of the neck until the chin comes close to the chest. Focusing the effort in the abdominal muscles, curl the shoulders off the floor towards the hips while breathing out. Do not let the lower back come off the floor. If the exercise is done properly, you will notice the lower back being pressed onto the floor increasingly harder as the movement progresses. This shows the role of the abdominal muscles in flattening the lumbar curve when they are tightened. Once you have curled up as far as you can, hold the final position for a second or two, lower yourself back to the floor, and breathe in. As soon as your head touches the floor, begin the next repetition. If you find that the body's weight is too great, fold your hands across your chest and try again. If this is still too difficult, hold your arms out straight, by your sides. Work up to doing ten repetitions. Remember to do the exercise sufficiently slowly so that each increment of movement is produced by a contraction of the relevant muscle—never use momentum to lift yourself up.

In the first few weeks of practicing the movement, the main effects may well be felt in the front neck muscles. This is because these muscles are weak in most people with sedentary lifestyles—and isn't that most of us these days? So, if your neck muscles tire *before* your stomach muscles while

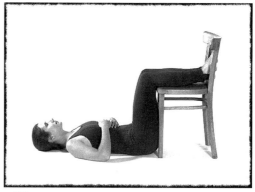

3

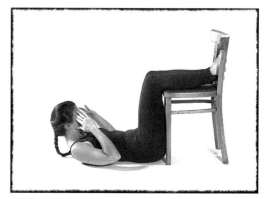

2

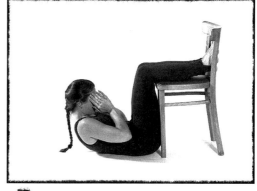

1

Notes

fingers *next* to temples

breathe out, and

very slowly lift head and curl body

don't lift lower back from floor

breathe in as you return to floor

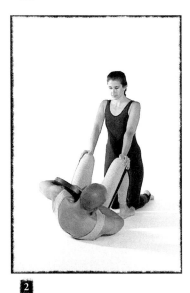

1

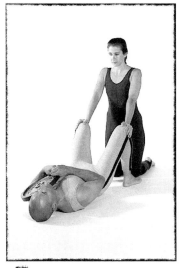

2

Notes

breathe out, and

while aiming face to *one* leg,

curl neck and body *slowly*

hold at top of position for count of "one, two"

breathe in while returning to floor

repeat for other side

practicing the movement, you may support the head with your arms for a few extra repetitions in order to do more work with the abdominals. In time, the front neck muscles will become sufficiently strong that you will start to feel the effects of the exercise in the abdominal muscles after you take the exercise to failure. Remember, the neck muscles stand in the same relation to the posterior neck muscles as the abdominals do to the extensor muscles of the lumbar spine; and they need to be reasonably strong. We have found that strengthening the neck muscles in this simple way has beneficial effects on many kinds of neck problems.

You may increase the resistance of the movement when ten repetitions can be done easily. Hold a small weight against your forehead (a book will do in the beginning), and otherwise all directions remain the same. Make sure that you are lifting the weight with the forehead (it is easy to cheat by lifting the weight with the hands). The effect on the front neck muscles will be intensified, but they will adapt quickly, and the extra resistance will make the abdominals stronger.

The basic crunch can be done slightly differently to produce an additional effect. In the **asymmetric version**, the resistance weight is held against one shoulder and the curling movement is performed *towards the opposite hip*. This means that in addition to the abdominal muscles at the front of the trunk, the *obliques* and the rib muscles on one side are also affected, as they contract to raise that shoulder higher as the trunk curls. Most people doing this version of the exercise exaggerate the movement by inclining their trunks too far outside the midline of the body. The exercise should be done twice; the second time with the weight on the other shoulder. Because the abdominal muscles work wherever the weight is positioned, start the exercise with the weight on one shoulder one session, and on the other shoulder in the next exercise session. Over time, the net effect will be balanced. Although shown on the floor, this movement may also be done on an inclined board (with the feet held higher than the head), affecting the lower abdominal muscles to a greater degree in most people.

The exercise may also be performed without a weight, by placing the hands together palm to palm at one side of the face and inclining the face to the hip on that side (then changing hand position and doing the other side), or by placing the fingers at the temples (as the first version described above) and alternating the inclination from side to side. If you decide to do the side-to-side version, alternate the movement until you can no longer complete a full contraction to one side, then finish the exercise by doing as many slow repetitions of the standard crunch as you can.

35. Abdominal curl over support

The exercise is shown over a purpose-built support. We use "barrels" made from 5-gallon drums cut lengthwise, with four legs and internal bracing. They can also be made from 44-gallon drums, for larger or less flexible people. You may be able to make something similar, or ask a welding shop to do the job. This "low-tech" approach gives excellent results for both stretching and strengthening exercises.

The curved surface ensures that the contraction of the abdominal muscles is progressive, and through a much wider range of movement than in the floor abdominal exercise detailed above. Depending on your flexibility, the range of movement could be double. An additional benefit of working on a curved surface is that we can smoothly change the angle through which we want the muscles to work, and the part of the spine in contact with the surface of the barrel is supported. Finally, changing the start position changes the angle of the body in relation to gravity, and hence changes the force curves generated in the muscles. Although you may not have such objects lying around the house, a little ingenuity will locate a substitute.

Look at the sequence of photographs. Note the way the body is stretching over the barrel in the first frame. Lower yourself into this position slowly and relax there for a moment to stretch. Make sure that you do this over a curvature which is suitable for you (not too small a radius). A larger support is better than a small one at first. When you attempt this for the first time, do not allow yourself to go back as far as you think you can. Rather, cautiously let yourself go back part of the way only. Then curl your head towards your chest to initiate the movement, and begin lifting your shoulders off the support, trying (as in the abdominal curl) to curl up into as tight a ball as possible. Do not try to lift your lower back from the support, because this will engage the hip flexors. The next time you lower yourself to the starting position, let yourself go down a little further; after a few repetitions let yourself go down as far as you can. In this way the initial repetitions become your warmup. The need to do the movement slowly cannot be overemphasized—each increment of forward movement must be by muscle contraction alone and not by momentum. Try to work up to doing ten slow repetitions. As with the abdominal curl, breathe in as you stretch backwards, and out as you curl up.

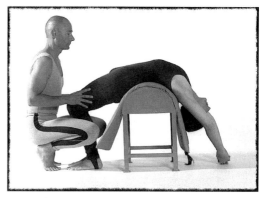

Stretch first

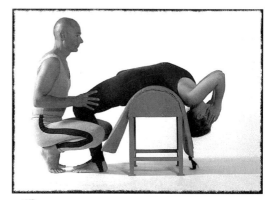

1

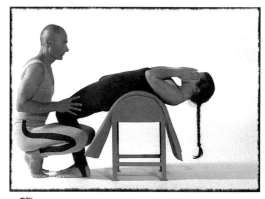

2 Very slowly curl neck and body

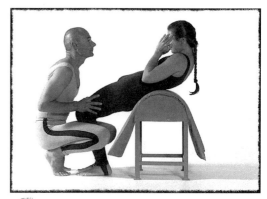

3

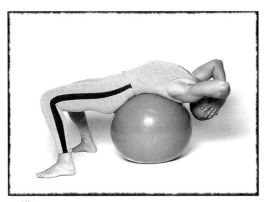

4

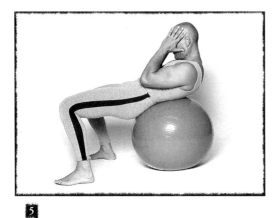

5

Notes

feet apart for stability

fingers next to temples, breathe out, and

slowly lift head; slowly curl body up

hold at top position

breathe in, return, and stretch back over ball

This exercise may be intensified by using a small weight, as with the floor abdominal crunch. If you do use a weight (a book or similar object), do not be surprised if you feel the main effects in the muscles of the front of the neck for the first few weeks.

The second sequence shows the same movement, but over an exercise ball, mentioned in exercise 28. These balls are commonly used in fitness classes around the world. I believe that stretching backwards over a firm padded support has advantages for postural rehabilitation, as exercise balls tend to deform precisely where your back has restrictions in its extension. Another disadvantage is that their unstable surface discourages relaxing in the stretch position, the very condition we have found so necessary in order to achieve a maximum stretch. In fact, the instability in this position can lead to muscle cramping in back pain sufferers. However, for advanced strengthening work these same aspects become significant advantages. Exercising abdominal muscles in an unstable environment maximizes the involvement of groups of muscles which act as stabilizers of parts of the skeleton, fixing one part to allow other muscles to do work. Some recent research suggests that weakness in *multifidus* (a lumbar spine muscle) and *transversus abdominis* (one of the abdominal muscles) plays a role in low back pain. Exercising over an unstable ball will maximize their involvement in the curling movement. You may care to experiment with different pressures in the ball too. As with the firm support described above, the strength requirement in particular parts of the range of movement will change as your position over the ball changes. Increasing the variety of the demands made of the muscles will maximize adaptation in strength and proprioception.

36. Back uncurl

A familiar strengthening exercise for the back muscles involves lying face-down with the arms in a suitable position, determined by one's strength. The head and shoulders are lifted from the floor by arching the back, and in some versions the legs are also lifted. One problem with this exercise is that the muscles will be doing work outside their normal functional range of movement.

The demands of normal daily life are to straighten a bent back. In the exercise just described, the muscles are required to hyperextend an already straight spine further backwards to an arched position. The risk of irritating structures involved in the original back pain is considerable. The pain may be muscular in origin or the result of compression of the joints of the spine. There is a very real risk of the muscles involved becoming cramped by this demand, or going into spasm—just because they are being asked to do work outside their normal range of movement. Any muscle working outside its normal range of movement is likely to cramp, if the demand is made in the strongly contracted part of its range. The final problem is one of specificity, a principle of strength training. Muscles respond by becoming stronger in the range of movement trained. Any strength gains made in the hyperextended range using the standard exercise are unlikely to be useful in daily life activities.

The following exercise is designed to avoid these pitfalls. It demands effort from the back muscles in the range of movement required in daily life. The movement requires a padded bench, a firm cylindrical cushion, the wide padded end of a strong couch, or an exercise ball for more advanced versions. Any surface over which you can drape the body will do, providing it will support you safely. When attempting to strengthen the muscles of a "problem" back, it is better to have the whole spine supported. In this exercise, the whole spine is supported, and after some practice you will be able to work the back muscles through a wide range of movement.

Look at the photographs. The first sequence shows the exercise over a flat bench. Begin by lying face-down over the support. The hips are flexed and the whole body relaxed. The starting position is similar to the final position of the abdominal strengthening exercise, but upside down.

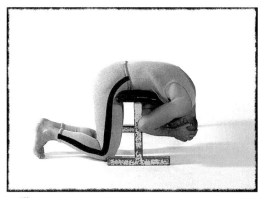

1

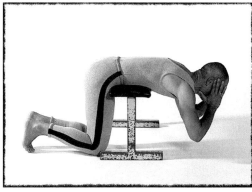

2 Stomach must press onto support

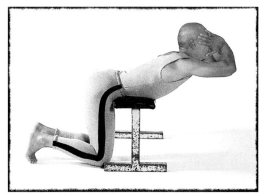

3

Notes

breathe *out* to get into start position

fingers next to temples

lead movement with head; breathe *in*

arch back; don't lift trunk from support

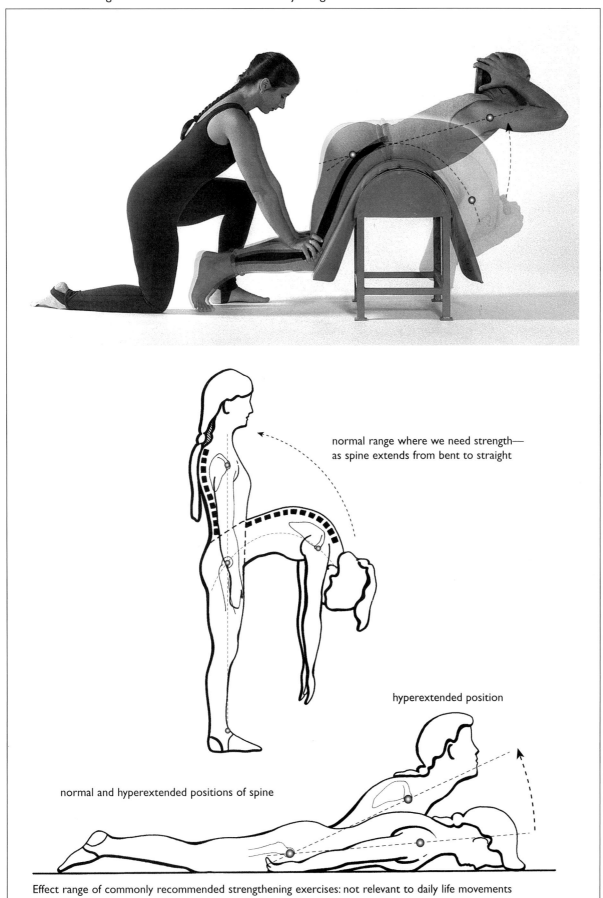

normal range where we need strength—
as spine extends from bent to straight

hyperextended position

normal and hyperextended positions of spine

Effect range of commonly recommended strengthening exercises: not relevant to daily life movements

This movement can be considered the reverse of the last exercise, strengthening the muscles on the other side of the trunk.

This exercise is called the back uncurl, to remind you of how it is to be done—you "peel" or "uncurl" the body off the support, beginning the movement with the head, progressively tightening upper, middle and lower back muscles in turn. Visualizing the action just before you try it will help you feel the right muscles and improve your action.

Place the fingertips against the temples and tuck the chin as close to the chest as you can; this flexes the spine forward. After lifting the head up, breathe in. Contract the muscles of the upper back, then those of the middle of the back, and finally those of the lower back. Do not lift the whole body off the support because this would involve the bottom muscles as well, and would take the body away from the support. Instead, just as you pressed the lower back into the floor in the abdominal exercise discussed in the previous section, you need to feel the support pressing quite hard into the lower abdominal area to be sure that the spine remains supported. You do not need to arch much above the point where the back is straight; in other words, do not hyperextend the spine. Breathe out as you lower yourself to the starting position. Note that breathing is not easy in this exercise because of the weight of the body on the abdominal area.

Look at the second sequence of photographs, where I am using a barrel for support. Always choose a support with a wide radius for your first attempts. If there are no adverse reactions, you can decrease the radius of the support so that the strengthening and stretching effects are experienced through a wider range. Remember, the smaller the radius, the greater the range through which the body can bend backwards and the stronger the effects will be.

Start by trying to do the movement as described. In the beginning, many people try to do the movement by lifting the whole body off the support, but this will not do. You need to uncurl; that is, the back muscles need to be contracted individually, from the uppermost (the neck muscles) all the way down to the lowest. Notice that although the neck muscles experience only the weight of the head, the resistance being applied to the muscles of the back increases as more of the body is lifted. This matches the

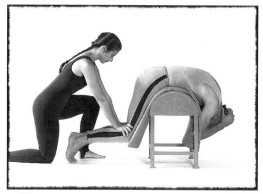

1

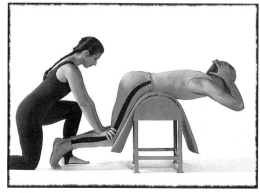

2 Stomach must press onto support

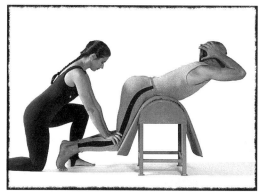

3

Notes

breathe *out* to get into start position
fingers next to temples
lead movement with head; breathe *in*
arch back; don't lift trunk from support
partner: hold back of knees

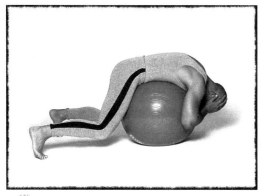

2 Feet apart for stability

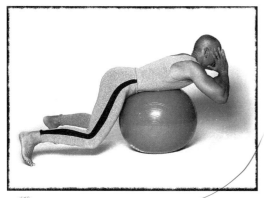

1

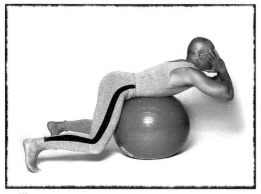

3

demands of daily life almost perfectly. Once you can do ten slow repetitions, you can use a small weight behind the neck—even a book will do. Breathe out as you return to the starting position, and breathe in as soon as you lift the head. Ensure that you do the movement slowly so that momentum does not help you. As with the abdominal exercises, every increment of movement must be the result of a greater force having been applied.

A partner may help as shown, by holding the back of the knees. The assistance is mainly to keep you on the same place on the support. Additionally, you will need a partner when the weight you are using lifts your feet from the floor as you contract the back muscles.

In the ball version of the exercise, one's body weight will be sufficient to begin—the increase in difficulty experienced compared to doing the exercise over a stable support is hard to imagine until you try. You will feel that a large number of additional muscles come into play in the unstable environment, and these stabilizer muscles are precisely the ones we need to strengthen. Experiment with varying the extension movement by adding a small rotation component, achieved by lifting one shoulder slightly higher than the other as you lift. Do an equal amount of work on both sides, comparing left with right.

Notes

focus on moving body symmetrically

movements *must* be slow

breathe in as you arch back

breathe out as you relax forwards

37. Trunk rotation

This movement and its variants are perhaps the most important strengthening exercises for the lower back you can do at home. Although included in the strengthening section, it is both a strengthening and a stretching exercise when performed to the extent of your range of movement. Additionally, if the source of your back pain is *quadratus lumborum* (refer to exercise 10 for details), this exercise done in its easiest form can ease the discomfort of a back pain attack considerably. No matter what your overall strength level, you must begin the exercise with minimum resistance (legs completely bent at the knees). Look at the first photograph. Notice that the hands are palm down, pressing on the floor. This stabilizes the shoulders, and holds them onto the floor. If your legs are relatively heavy, you will need to press quite hard to keep the shoulders on the floor. At this stage, the thighs are vertical, and the heels held near the bottom.

In the **easiest** version, lie as shown with the knees completely bent. Let your legs and hips roll to one side, *aiming the knees at one hand*. This instruction is vital to avoid hyperextending the spine, and essential to achieving the stretch in the lower back. Once you feel the weight of the legs (in the muscles of the waist and lower back), gently lower the legs as close to the floor as you can, keeping the knees aimed at the hand on that side. This is the stretch phase. Rest for a few breaths in and out in the final position. Then, with an exhalation, *slowly* lift the legs back up to the starting position by using the muscles of the waist. Of course, the muscles of the arms and shoulders will be working too, in a support role, but try as much as possible to use the muscles of the waist to lift the legs. This is the strengthening part. Repeat the movement several times with the legs in the completely bent position, from one side to the other.

Try not to rest the legs on the floor, because the muscles will not be working if you do. If you are flexible, you can keep the tension on the working muscles by briefly touching the floor with the knees at the end of the movement on each side and beginning the lifting phase immediately. We try to keep the tension on the muscles throughout the exercise to tire them as quickly as possible, one of the ways we use to keep the intensity high.

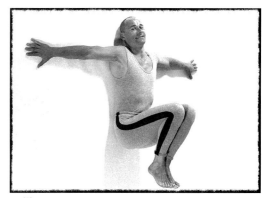

1 Easiest

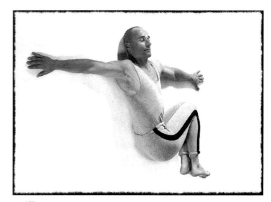

2

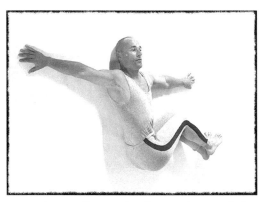

Intermediate version (legs partly extended)

If you can do this version with no discomfort, and are able to hold the shoulders against the floor, in the **intermediate** version you may increase both the stretch and the resistance by partially straightening the legs. Try to hold the knees together while doing the movement, but maintain the angle; that is, check that regardless of the position of the lower leg, the thighs are pointing at your hand.

Notes

press *palms* to floor to hold
shoulders to floor

breathe out as you lower legs
towards floor

tighten stomach muscles,
breathe out, and

slowly lift legs to start position

repeat for other side

Correct form in exercise 37

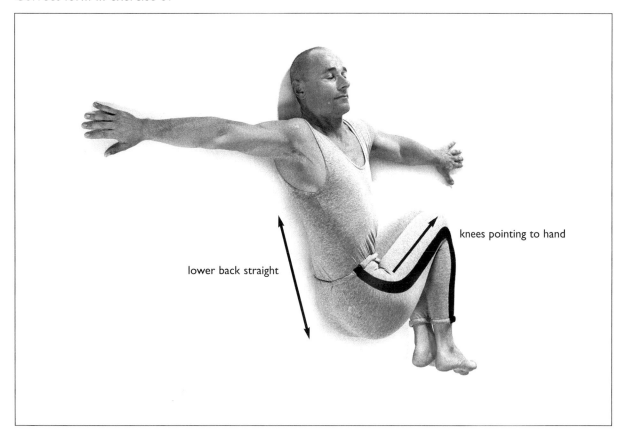

lower back straight

knees pointing to hand

The strongest stretch (and consequently the strongest resistance in the strengthening phase) is when you can hold the legs straight throughout the movement. This is an **advanced** exercise and you must work up to it slowly. Building up to the exercise at this level of difficulty could take many months. Do not sacrifice form to try to do the exercise with straight legs.

The first few times you do the movement, go from one side to the other in turn, comparing sides. Do not be surprised if you find that they are not symmetrical. Asymmetry is common, and something one expects to find, particularly in people with back problems. Asymmetry comes in two basic forms in this movement: one side less flexible, or one side weaker. First, determine what kind of imbalance you have: is one rotation direction tighter or is one direction weaker?

Choose the imbalance you wish to address. We can apply the appropriate balancing stress in one of two ways: if one side is tighter, emphasize the stretch aspect on that side when you next do the exercise, by holding the stretch position for a few seconds at each end point of a repetition. If one side is weaker, we can emphasize the strengthening aspect by doing the work only on that side to begin with. Let us say, for argument's sake, that you were able to do nine repetitions in good form on the weak side. Repeat the exercise now on the stronger side, but do only as many repetitions as you were able to do for the first side. Doing so will be easier of course. The effect over time will be to stress the weaker side significantly more than the other, so that it will respond more quickly. Eventually both sides will be similar, if not the same. As a general rule, for any exercise one can do for one side of the body, the upper limit of repetitions or weight handled should be the same as what can be handled by the weaker or less flexible side. For strengthening, it is preferable to work one side at a time because the muscles have far less time to rest between contractions, and increasing intensity increases rate of adaptation.

Do not do too many of these movements initially. This is a very strong exercise, and you will need to work up to it slowly. As with the stretching movements, err on the side of doing too little in the beginning. For women, developing the requisite arm and shoulder strength may be the limiting factor in the first instance.

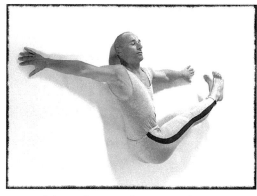

Advanced version (legs straight)

Breathing in a particular way can help you in this exercise. Breathe in while the legs are vertical, and hold the breath as you lower the legs. Breathe out as you lift the legs. When holding the breath, do not take in a deeper breath than normal. By not breathing out during the lowering phase you will achieve two things: the trunk is made stronger by the Valsalva maneuver maneuver (the compression of the abdominal contents by the muscles of the trunk); and the exhalation makes you a little stronger in the exertion phase. Do not exaggerate these suggestions.

Although described as a trunk rotation exercise, the main strengthening effects will be experienced in the lower trunk, especially the muscles that stabilize the pelvis. The upper trunk muscles and the muscles of the arms and shoulders are used mainly to stabilize the upper body so the lower trunk muscles can do their work.

38. *Trunk rotation with weight*

This movement helps strengthen the waist muscles, but can be made much more intense than the previous exercise and it can work through a wider range of movement. This is also an excellent stretching exercise, if you are tight in rotation, since the maximum effect of the weight is experienced at the extremes of the range of the movement.

Begin your first attempt with a light weight (for women 5–10 lb.; for men 10–20 lb.), holding it at arms' length as shown. Imagine that the weight is a mirror—as you do the movement, imagine that you are trying to keep your face in view. If you are able to do this, you will be maintaining the weight and your chest in the correct alignment. Because we are handling the weight to strengthen the waist muscles, it is essential that every increment of movement at the hands is due to a *rotation* of the waist rather than a movement of the arms and shoulders with respect to the body. Think of the exercise in this way: the arms and chest form a rectangle with the weight, and this complex (weight, arms, chest) is moved as one unit by the waist and back muscles. Look at the photographs carefully—these details are important if you want to gain maximum benefit from the exercise.

Hold the weight, and visualize rotating only at the waist. Let the weight (together with the arms and chest) move across and sink towards the floor, slowly. If you are successful in not letting the arms move with respect to the chest, your shoulders will be close to vertical if you are flexible enough to lower the weight to the floor. Feel the stretch. Ideally, this should be felt in the muscles of the lower back, on the side you are turning away from (now the upper side). Being aware of where you feel the stretch, slowly lift the weight back to the starting position *using the stretched muscles*. I suggest breathing in as the weight is brought to the midline of the body each repetition.

We have found in the gym that people use two ways to get the weight to the floor: rolling over *on* the shoulder (producing a slight straightening of the spine, and which emphasizes *quadratus lumborum* in the movement) and rolling the shoulder *under* as the movement progresses (which distributes the effort over more of the trunk muscles). Try both and see which you prefer. If you are training on your own, you will need to fix the feet under a strong support, because the *hip flexors* and the leg muscles

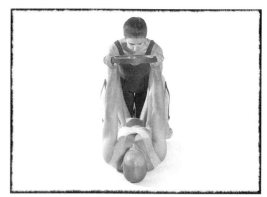

1

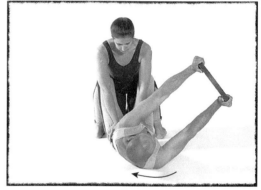

2   Draw shoulder *under*

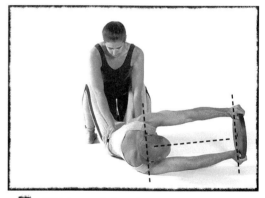

3   Weight parallel to chest

Notes

pretend the weight is a mirror

tighten stomach muscles
as you exert

breathe normally

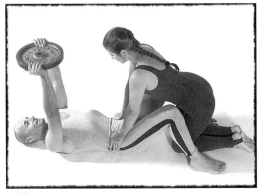

1

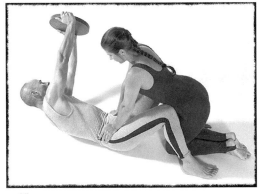

2 Rolling *on* shoulder

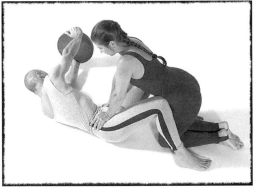

3

will be drawn upon to hold the pelvis in position as the weight held in the arms increases. Do not let the hips come off the floor.

The side that feels the weaker or less flexible (that is, does not go as close to the floor) must determine how many repetitions are done for the other side. You need to find out which side has the lesser capacity (of either strength or flexibility) and do only that number of repetitions for the other side too. This will ensure that the weaker or tighter side will catch up with the other because it is experiencing the greater stimulus for change.

In the first few weeks, women may find that the main strengthening effects from the exercise will be felt in the arms rather than the trunk muscles; this is normal. As the arm and shoulder muscles become stronger, women will be able to use more weight, and consequently greater effects will be felt in the trunk. For any athlete whose sport demands the transfer of the strength of one half of the body to the other (essential in golf or rowing, for example) this exercise should be the cornerstone of your strengthening routine. In our gym classes, we have found that spending a few weeks strengthening the trunk (and also the arms, for women) allows the trainee to acquire whole-body strength in the compound exercises significantly faster than fellow trainees who start their programs with the compound exercises, as is usually done. A strong trunk is essential in daily life.

Notes

pretend the weight is a mirror

partner must hold hips to floor

ADVANCED STRENGTHENING EXERCISE (PREVENTION)

39. Knee lift

This is the premier abdominal muscle strengthening exercise. In its advanced form it is also the most difficult of the abdominal movements. You must not attempt even the easiest form of this exercise until you can do ten or more slow repetitions of the abdominal curl described in exercise 34. Do the knee lift with a partner, so he or she can check your form and help you in the assistance positions if desired. Attention to form is essential, as the effectiveness of the knee lift movement is easy to circumvent, and one can see this exercise being done in poor form in gyms anywhere around the world.

In this final exercise, I wish to introduce another way to increase the intensity of any exercise, which you will recall is the main determinant of the extent of the adaptive response. In the strengthening exercises described so far, we have been using *concentric* strength building movements; that is, we have been shortening the muscles against a resistance. In *eccentric* strength exercises you demand work of the muscles by making them *resist elongation* by a force or weight. Such repetitions are usually called "negatives." Any weight training exercise can be done in this way, but there are a few disadvantages. One is that you will generally need a partner to help you do the work during the concentric phase (the partner will need to help you move the weight or the body to a starting position from which you will lower it), because the body is about 40–50% stronger in eccentric movements than in concentric ones. This means that you will need to be handling significantly heavier resistance than you would normally, with consequently greater risk of injury and greater muscle soreness following training. Some researchers claim this increased soreness is because the junctions between tendons and their muscles take more of the strain than they do in concentric training; others claim the increased soreness is a result of the greater proportion of muscle fibers recruited in any repetition.

Nonetheless, some exercises lend themselves very well to negative training, and the various forms of the hanging knee lift are perfect examples. It is worth mentioning at this point that although negative training is not used as often as

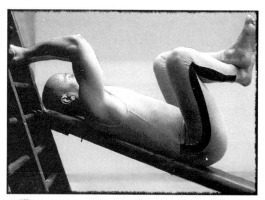

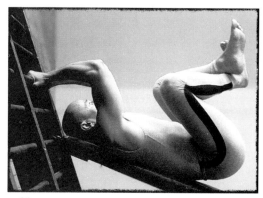

1   Easiest version

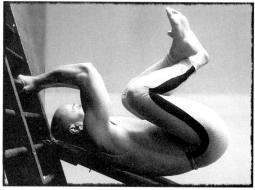

2

3

Notes

lift knees until hips move (start)

on breath out, *slowly* draw
knees to chest

upper back must stay on board

hold finish position for two count

breathe in, and slowly lower

concentric exercise in the weight training gym, it is the most commonly used method for teaching strength moves in gymnastics. Negative training simply involves lowering a weight that is too heavy to lift normally, in a slow and controlled way. The negative phase of the movement should take three to five seconds, depending on momentum considerations and the range of movement involved—the greater the range, the more time it should take.

The knee lift requires lifting the knees as closely as possible to the chest. Many of you may recognize the movement from the gym, but this version has been modified in significant ways. In the conventional form, you hang from a bar or from an elbow support with the legs hanging down. The legs are then swung up; one version letting the knees bend, and the other keeping the legs straight. The problem with both these versions is similar to the problems with conventional sit-ups—the powerful hip flexors move the legs in the first 90 degrees (or more) of the knee lift and the resulting momentum completes the movement. To see why this is significant, stand on one leg with one hand feeling the abdominal muscles. Lift one knee up to about horizontal, and you will find that the stomach muscles in fact do not contract at all. Even when the knees are lifted together, the hip flexors do most of the work in the first 90 degrees of movement. This means the exercise, as it is normally done, will not strengthen the abdominal muscles as is claimed.

The **easiest** version of this exercise requires an adjustable incline board. I have shown this movement on an incline board that uses a set of "ladder bars" for its support. Look at the photographs. I am holding the ladder bars with a supinated (palms facing shoulders) grip, as the arm muscles are in their strongest positions this way. If you do not have access to ladder bars, hold the edges of the incline board itself above your head to stabilize the upper body. To find your starting position, slowly lift the legs with the knees bent as close to your chest as you can, *without lifting the body*. You will reach a point where any further movement of the knees towards the chest will lift the hips off the board. This indicates the starting position. Note that a combination of hip flexibility and muscle attachments will result in different starting positions for each person. Typically, women's starting positions will have the knees closer to their chests than men's. Some people can bring their knees all the way back to their chests without lifting the body from the support. If this is the case, you will need to have the knees far enough apart so that when you do the exercise you can take the knees *past* the body, under the arms.

From the starting position, the exercise is done by slowly lifting the knees towards (or past) the chest until the abdominal muscles are fully contracted. This is done by telling yourself to bring the knees closer to the chest (or past the body, depending on your start position). *The upper back must stay on the support surface* if you wish to avoid a common fault—lifting the whole body off the board with the strength of the arm and back muscles. Each contraction increment of the abdominal muscles must produce a change in the shape of the spine, from straight (the starting position) to curved (the fully contracted, finish position). To be sure, have your partner check your form. Stop lifting when the middle and upper back begins to lift off the board. Do not use a sudden movement of the knees to generate momentum to achieve the movement, which is the most common fault. Slower is better here—as you will quickly feel. Adjust the incline to a steeper angle as you become stronger.

Your partner may help in the following ways. For the first month or two, ask your partner to assist you to complete a few additional repetitions after you no longer can complete repetitions by yourself, by pressing lightly on your feet and taking a *small* amount of the weight of the legs. This assistance should be the least required effort—when you fail to complete a repetition, you are failing with that *specific* resistance; and if it is reduced even slightly, you will be able to do further work. When you feel ready, you can extend this "failure zone" by asking your partner to add "negatives" after you have completed the assisted positives described. Have your partner lift the knees to or past the chest; your partner then lets the knees go, and you will try to hold them there. After a second or so, take four to five seconds to lower the legs to the starting position. Repeat this for a few additional repetitions.

To attempt the **advanced** version, you will need to hang vertically from a support bar, either from your arms, or from arm supports (straps that are looped over the bar and support you under the upper arm, to save you hanging from your hands). The first task is to determine your own start position. Have your partner stand to one side of you to observe the shape of your lower back. Lift your knees up until your partner informs you that your lower back is just starting to change shape from its normal backwards curve to straight. This indicates that the abdominal muscles are beginning to contract. This is your start position, and in each subsequent repetition you must not let the legs drop lower than this. Slowly lift the knees as close to the chest as you can (or past the arms if necessary), taking a few seconds to complete the movement. Hold the knees up in this position, and count "one, two" to yourself. Lower under control to your start position, and repeat. You will need to breathe out as you lift the knees.

Let us assume that you were able to do a few repetitions before no longer being able to lift the knees from the start position, even trying hard. Now we use the negative approach. Ask your partner to lift the knees as close to the chest as possible, and you try to hold them there. Hold the position for a second or two if you can, and then slowly lower the knees to your starting position. Immediately, have your partner lift the knees back to the chest. Again, you hold and then slowly lower them. As the muscles become more fatigued, your capacity to lower your legs slowly decreases, and the legs fall to the starting position more and more quickly. As soon as you cannot control the lowering (and the knees drop as soon as your partner lets them go), stop. Try only a few of these "negatives" the first time you attempt the exercise—if you do too many of them your stomach muscles will be sore for *days*. Make haste slowly. If you are not able to do negatives with the full weight of the legs, have your partner take some of the weight and try hard to control the remainder.

Always breathe out strongly as you lift the knees (full lungs will hinder the completion of the movement) and breathe in as you lower the legs. Because this exercise is strenuous, you may find that you need extra breaths in and out during each repetition, especially if you are working negatively. Breathe where it feels most natural.

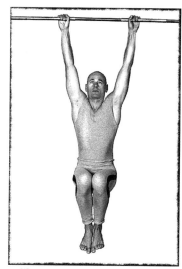

1 Advanced version

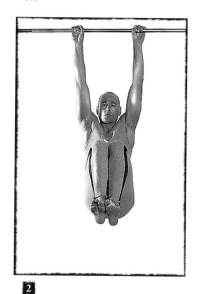

2

Notes

partner lifts knees to start position

slowly lift knees close to chest

try to hold position for two count

slowly lower legs *until back is straight*

breathe, and repeat

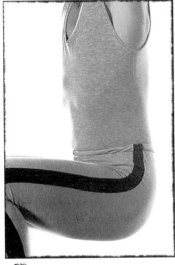

1

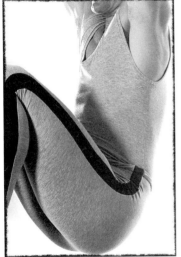

2 The shape of the spine *must* change if the abdominal muscles are doing the work

Notes

lift knees *slowly*

bring knees closer to body

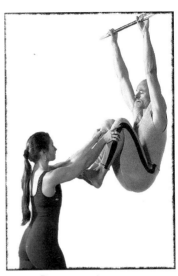

Doing negatives

Notes

partner lifts knees to chest

hold the knees in position for two count

slowly lower knees under control

don't hold your breath

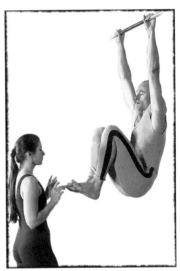

2

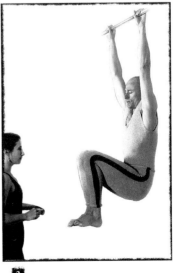

3

One of the reasons this movement is so successful is that the whole upper body is stretched in the starting position. When you lift the knees to the chest in this exercise, many muscles are involved besides the complex of abdominal muscles. The muscles in between the ribs (*intercostals*), the back muscles under the arms, and the arm muscles themselves are all at work, just trying to hang onto the bar.

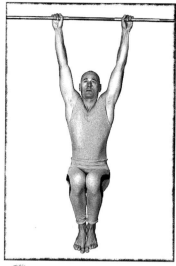

When you feel confident with the movement, ask your partner to stand to one side and watch you do it. If you are doing it correctly, the normal lumbar curve should flatten, then round out as you complete the exercise. The abdominal muscles span the ribs and the pubic bones, so that if they are shortening the shape of the lumbar curve will change. Recall that it is possible for someone with good hip flexibility to lift the knees very close to the chest using only the hip flexors. When you can do ten concentric repetitions, your abdominal muscles will be very strong indeed.

In the final **advanced** version of the exercise, lift one hip higher than the other as you lift the knees up to the chest. This will affect the side waist muscles (*obliques*) as well as the abdominals, and the muscles in between the ribs (*intercostals*) on the side you are lifting towards. This movement must be done slowly to be effective; that is, take a few seconds at least to complete one repetition—first to one side then to the other. To reduce the strain of hanging from the bar for too long, you can do the repetitions for one side, get down off the bar and rest, and do the repetitions for the other side a little later. To make sure the waist muscles develop evenly over time if you follow this latter suggestion, begin with the left side on one training day, and on the next training day begin with the right side. Breathing is the same as for the previous versions.

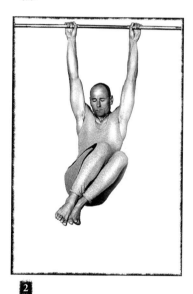

This completes the elements of my approach to overcoming neck and back pain. Let us now turn our attention to the integration of these various elements.

Notes

draw knee to opposite shoulder

lift *slowly*, on breath out

hold top position for two count

lower and straighten
to start position

use *only* trunk muscles
to curl body

PLANNING A TOTAL ROUTINE

Frequency of exercise

You do not need to do anywhere near as much exercise as most experts say. As I mentioned at the beginning of the strengthening section, most people who start an exercise program abandon it within a month or six weeks. The main reason for this is that they have embarked on a program that is far too ambitious for their needs or (perhaps more significantly) their capacity. For a program to endure, and to be enjoyable—an essential aspect for any long-term prospects of sticking with it—it must fit your lifestyle. Moreover, despite the near-crippling exercise regimens your favorite athlete grinds through each day or week, your needs are not the same. Our goal is to optimize health, with an emphasis on rectifying, or preventing, neck and back pain.

Having said this, two Australian National women rowers I once coached trained with weights only twice a week for 30–40 minutes a session. This was complemented by two 10–15 minute stretching sessions each week, the stretching being done after the weight training. Their training involved only one set of each of seven exercises, some of these requiring a warmup set. Each set was performed to complete failure; that is, until they were temporarily incapable of further repetitions, or even partial repetitions, of the movement. Their performance over a twelve-month period improved faster than that of their fellow crew members, all of whom were doing three one-hour weight training sessions a week, each involving the usual three to five maximum sets, but with no stretching. The work capacities of these athletes is tested periodically by using an ergometer, a rowing machine that measures power output.

The point of this story is that the *quality* of your training is a significant determinant of improvement, and for beginners is more important than is the amount of weight handled, the numbers of "sets" (work groups of repetitions) and "reps" (repetitions), or the total amount of work done (training volume). Nautilus Foundation research has suggested that the old adage "less is more" may be correct, as far as weight training is concerned, provided there is genuine maximum intensity in the effort. In conventional training the maximum intensity the body experiences with respect to any exercise usually occurs during the final few repetitions of the last set. If the research into determinants of adaptation is correct, the body responds to the stimulation of just those last repetitions—any previous sets' repetitions (because you were not exhausting yourself doing them) are more or less a waste of time. It should be noted, however, that beginners to weight training will make improvements on almost any system. What I am interested in pursuing here is: How can one get the fastest results for the least amount of time spent?

The multiple-set approach to most weight training should be avoided by people wishing to rehabilitate themselves for neck or back problems, for a number of reasons. Firstly, following a warmup, if you know that there are three or five work sets to be done, you cannot help saving yourself for the later sets. This has two consequences. The first is that maximum intensity is experienced either in the last few repetitions of the last set, or not experienced at all. Instead, you tend to work at about 80% of your possible capacity, doing a lot of work, but at suboptimal intensity. This is commonly observed in gyms everywhere. The second consequence is that any sets not experienced at your maximum merely use energy and nutrients that otherwise would be used to repair the body following the maximum intensity set. This suggests strongly that sets before or additional to the one at which the maximum intensity was experienced actually detract from the training response. This is even more likely to be so if you have a stressful life, because your capacity to adapt to the extra stress of the weight training is reduced. Furthermore, if you leave the gym knowing that you have worked at your maximum intensity yet also feeling that you have not exhausted yourself (that, in fact, you could do more work), your attitude to returning to the gym is positive and there is far less likelihood of overtraining or staleness. Overtraining can be a real danger, even for the weekend athlete. Faster progress in strength training goals will be realized if the suggested approach is followed, at least for the first year or so. This approach is much more efficient in terms of results gained for time spent. It is certainly more enjoyable.

The intensity of the experience seems to be the most important factor. Thus some specific recommendations can be made for your workouts, realizing that individual requirements or reactions will alter the details in each case. Indeed, the shape and emphasis of your routine should change over time to reflect changing priorities and your improvement.

Sets and reps

The number of times you repeat a movement is referred to as the number of repetitions, or "reps." Groups of repetitions (from beginning to when you can do no more) are referred to as "sets." How many sets, of how many reps, should one do? Before making a specific recommendation, let us explore the standard approaches.

The conventional suggestions range from a standard of three sets of about ten repetitions per body part to the serious bodybuilder's eight to twenty sets, with the repetitions varying from five to eight (or from ten to fifteen), depending on the desired outcome. For a bodybuilder, the choice is said to depend on whether one is working in a strengthening phase (to get stronger and to put on muscle weight) or a refining phase (to bring out the shape of muscles). Others suggest that the number of sets and repetitions depends on whether you are seeking strength or endurance. Strength is said to be achieved by larger numbers of low-repetition sets (for example, ten sets of one to five reps, typical of Olympic lifting, for example), and endurance by smaller numbers of sets, but with much higher repetitions (for example, three sets of 25 to 35 repetitions, common among rowers). In the low-repetition, heavy-weight approach, the neurological system must adapt strongly in addition to the muscles, tendons and ligaments. Proprioception and coordination adaptations are emphasized by the near maximum weights handled. Adaptation to the high repetition, relatively small resistance approach occurs as much in the circulatory system as the muscle system, and when combined with very small resistances is used in fitness classes, where it is said to promote "toning" of the muscles.

However, my suggestions are different. If you have a need to demonstrate maximum one-repetition strength levels (as competitive weight lifters do, for example) then you need to follow a program which develops maximum strength in the whole structure and enables you to become familiar with handling weights which are close to your maximum for psychological and technical reasons. The emphasis will be as much on maximizing the neurological aspects (the extent to which you can mobilize the largest *numbers* of muscle fibers in maximum contractions) as in building strength in individual fibers. The dangers are obvious—the closer one is working to one's limit, the harder the exercise is to control, and the greater the possibility of injury. For this last reason alone, the maximum-strength-developing regime is not suitable for most of us. Neither is the high-repetition endurance system, but for different reasons. We are not particularly interested in developing specific muscle endurance. This type of training is also relatively tiring, and the high repetitions are not conducive to concentrating on perfect form, which is the top priority. This approach is also obviously unsuitable for anyone suffering from any kind of repetitive strain injury.

Because most of the strength exercises recommended in this book are done using the body's weight as resistance, the recommendations about selection of weight to be handled may seem somewhat academic. However, the principles as they relate to creation of the intensity effect remain relevant, and most can be implemented directly.

Taking account of the research on the different sets and reps approaches, it is best to err on the side of caution in the beginning, and attempt an exercise with a lighter weight than you imagine you might be able to handle, and concentrate on attaining good form. *Good form* must always remain the first priority. As mentioned, in some of the exercises you may not be able to do a single repetition with your body's weight—if so, get your partner to help and do the negative version. I recommend only one set of each exercise.

When you can do 15 repetitions of the movement, increase the weight—but only to one which permits a minimum of eight repetitions. The initial repetitions in the set will constitute a sufficient warmup, but the final four or five repetitions will be at maximum effort. In exercises using body weight, the weight which you will add may be very light and yet provide a significant additional resistance. For example, if you initially do the hanging knee lifting movement without shoes, it will take some time before you can do 15 repetitions. When that day comes, do the exercise with your shoes on. Although relatively light, the addition of this weight is significant because of the leverage factors (the length of thighs).

However, even following this prescription will not provide the ideal intensity for some exercises. How then can you follow the prescription and further increase intensity? The answer is to employ the principles of resistance reduction, assisted repetitions, negative repetitions and partial repetitions to your one set, singly or in combination.

Resistance reduction ("strip sets" or "drop sets" in gym speak) means that you reduce the weight by a small amount as soon as you feel that you will be unable to complete another full repetition without assistance. For example, assume that you are doing a barbell exercise with 100 lb. Thinking ahead, you will have made this weight up with two 20 lb. plates, and four 10 lb. plates (assuming 20 lb. bar). As soon as you feel that you are failing or losing the form, put the weight back on the stands. Ask your partner to take two 10 lb. plates off and recommence the exercise at once. These weight recommendations are a guide only—depending on the exercises you will need to have the increments smaller or larger. This approach can be applied to body's weight exercises (once you are using extra weight) by dropping the weight when you have tired, and continuing with body weight alone. In the exercises using plates, make up the total weight you require with two smaller ones.

Assisted repetitions are another way to prolong the repetitions at maximum effort. They can be used with either concentric or eccentric movements. Some exercises lend themselves to this technique in virtue of their physical arrangements—assistance is easier to give in some exercises than others. For example, to assist in the hanging knee lift movement, your partner waits until you can no longer perform another movement in good form. Then (by placing his or her palms under your feet or supporting the front of the knees) your partner takes a small amount of the weight of your legs as you try to lift them. Even reducing the weight of your legs by a tiny amount will enable you to do more repetitions. After all, muscle failure occurs when the force the muscles can apply only just fails to overcome the resistance. Reducing the resistance by even a small amount can let the muscles continue to work. In this way, the point of imminent failure—the very intensity I have been stressing throughout—can be prolonged for five or more repetitions beyond the point at which you would have otherwise stopped.

The term negative repetitions (*eccentric* contractions, or negatives for short) was used previously when discussing how to do an exercise you could not do positively (*concentrically*). This approach can also be used to prolong the maximum effort phase of any exercise, after you have done as many repetitions as possible in the positive phase. For example, assume you have done your nonassisted repetitions in the hanging knee lift exercise. Have your partner immediately lift your knees to your chest. Try to hold them there for an instant. As you feel yourself weakening, lower the knees slowly—a good negative repetition should take about four seconds—and fight the resistance all the way to the starting position. Again, before you have any chance to rest, have your partner lift your knees and let them go as soon as they reach your chest. Finish the exercise when you cannot prevent your knees from falling to the start position. Generally, this will require about five repetitions. This is very high intensity work indeed, so do not be in too much of a hurry to progress to this technique—it will leave the muscles very sore.

To experience the maximum in intensity, negative repetitions can even be added to an exercise after you have done a number of assisted repetitions (assisted in the positive phase) for an even greater effect. However, do not attempt this until you are completely confident with the assisted approach. Adding the negatives to the assisted method is extremely intense, and must not be attempted by anyone who has even a hint of their previous problems remaining.

Partial repetitions are unsuccessful attempts to complete full repetitions. The partial repetition that results is both *isotonic* (while the weight is still moving) and *isometric* (the point at which the weight no longer moves, no matter how hard you try). Partial repetitions can be used as a variation on combinations of the above elements, such as when you do not feel like progressing into the negative phases (for example, if you do not have a training partner, or do not feel like pushing yourself too hard). The hanging knee lift is a good example of an exercise that can be done in a variety of ways, by combining these different elements.

Working habits

As mentioned previously, many people begin training programs and give up after a short time. In addition to embarking on programs that are unsuitable or too ambitious, some of these people drop out because they fail to take into account personal lifestyle factors, such as children or the demands of work. For example, it is impossible to do your stretching exercises with your baby crawling all over you, and very unlikely that you will even feel like exercising after a 14-hour day at work. Part of the success of any exercise program is to choose the right time and the right location for your exercise, and not to take on too much.

The best time to stretch is in the late afternoon or evening before you have your evening meal, when the body is at its loosest. Stretching *after* weight training (or aerobic training) is ideal, as the muscles are warmest then. Although strengthening exercises can be done at any time, for someone getting over an injury it is best to avoid the mornings because the body is at its tightest. However, if you are a morning person, and you warmup carefully, then (presupposing that you are free of injuries) begin with the strengthening exercises and finish with the stretching exercises. Avoid doing strengthening exercises at night too soon before you sleep because they tend to stimulate the body and this may affect your sleep.

Any strength training or aerobic training is a perfect warmup for stretching—just try to keep as much of the generated body heat in the muscles by wearing appropriate clothes. The secret to maintaining a successful program is to integrate it as seamlessly as possible into your normal routine. This may indicate lunchtime training sessions, or before or after work. Use a facility that is close to either your house or work place to minimize inconvenience and wasted time.

If time constraints (or children) make these suggestions impracticable, you can still do the stretching exercises on the lounge room floor while watching television, after the children have gone to bed. Alternatively, it is a lot of fun to do these exercises with your children if they are old enough, and it is never too early to teach good habits.

Speed of movements

The correct speed of movement is critical. We have already considered the speed of stretching and must now look at the speed of strengthening exercises. In the positive phase of any movement, each increment of movement of the resistance weight—whether an object or part of your body—must be achieved by muscular contraction, and not by momentum generated in an earlier part of the movement. This cannot be overemphasized, and as a principle is second only to the importance of form. Do not make the movements too slow, either. As a rough guide (remembering that this will depend on the nature of the exercise to an extent), a positive contraction exercise should take about two to three seconds to complete, and negatives about twice as long.

Do not pause too long in either the extended or contracted phase of a movement. Usually, the beginning or end points of an exercise are relatively easy to hold and as such provide a rest for the muscles. Remember that we are trying to fatigue the muscles in the *shortest* possible time, and that prolonging the exercise defeats this goal. Try to put your total concentration into each instant of the doing of an exercise—this increases its intensity and reduces the chance of injury.

The importance of rest

Do not train too much. All adaptation to stimulation occurs after training, not during it. Accordingly, to adapt as fast as possible you will need to ensure that you have adequate rest. Studies show that all stress causes effects in the body—good and bad stress—and that the effects of one kind of stress tend to compound with those of other kinds of stress. These studies also show that everyone has an innate capacity to handle stress, and that if this capacity is exceeded the body cannot adapt to new stress.

As far as the body is concerned, a new exercise program is just another stress. Examples of stress include your job (the stress of which is likely to vary, depending on what you are doing at any time), other training you may be involved in or any significant change to your normal routine. Accordingly, you may need to reduce your involvement in other stressing activities if you wish to adapt to the new stress as quickly as possible.

The place of aerobic exercise

Swimming is often recommended to help alleviate back pain. This recommendation is usually made on the assumption that, because swimming is an aerobic activity in which the body's weight is supported while it is horizontal, it is good for patients recovering or suffering from back pain. I believe that this advice needs some qualification—it depends the style of swimming you adopt. If you are a good freestyle swimmer who breathes to both sides, the recommendation is generally sound, and the gentle and supported flexion and extension of the spine while supported by the water yields beneficial results. This may be the result of a mechanical effect on the intervertebral discs that increases water imbibition by the disc nucleus and helps to restore disc height.

However, if you are not a good freestyle swimmer, and have to use breast stroke or another style, swimming can make your problems worse. This can be the result of the slight to moderate hyperextension of the lumbar spine, and the contraction in the back muscles required to hold the head out of the water. For people with neck pain this problem can be significant. Many patients with back problems have reported that swimming makes their complaints worse. Thus swimming should not be used early in the rehabilitation phase, unless you are a good swimmer and the activity does not irritate the problem. However, swimming is excellent aerobic activity that can help to keep back pain at bay once the back has returned to normal, and this activity has many other benefits besides.

Running is also an excellent aerobic activity, but has obvious drawbacks for sufferers of back pain. The whole weight of the body is carried on the legs, there can be some slight to significant compression of the lumbar region, there are mechanical shocks to the spine with each step and most people run on hard surfaces that tend to exacerbate these problems. These negative aspects are worsened if the patient is carrying excess body weight. If the patient is a long-term runner, there is also a strong likelihood that the muscles of the lower back, the groin and the hamstrings will be less flexible than average, and this can also exacerbate the back pain. For runners, the importance of assessing any possible leg-length differences cannot be overemphasized. In general, a person suffering from back pain should not run until the pain has reduced to a nonsignificant level.

Cycling can be quite comfortable for the sufferer of back pain. However, it is contraindicated for the patient with neck pain, depending on the style of cycling. Racing bikes place a strain on the back of the neck and the upper back, whereas mountain bikes generally deliver more road shock to the lower back but place less strain on the neck, due to the more upright riding position. The value in cycling, especially stationary cycling, is that you can effectively and safely warm up the muscles you need to stretch. If you wear the appropriate clothes you can retain much of this heat. Remember that an increase of just one degree in core muscle temperature can increase flexibility 15% or more, and when your body is tight every fraction of a per cent of flexibility is significant.

Other values in aerobic activity during the recovery phase include the general feeling of well being after exercise and maintenance of your desired body weight. This encourages an optimistic frame of mind. All these factors have a bearing on a successful recovery.

Lifting things in everyday life

Before ending this chapter on strengthening techniques, we should look at how to avoid injuries while lifting. The most common history of patients with acute back pain, and the most common prelude to disc prolapse, is an unexceptional lifting movement done around the house or work place that combines extension with rotation. No such movement has been included in the strengthening exercises presented, with good reason.

A typical movement that combines rotation with extension is the action of picking up a trash can which is on the ground to one side of you. You not only bend forwards, but also rotate to one side. To pick up the can, you must lift with the legs, and lift and twist with the waist muscles. This can place large, nonsymmetrical forces on both the intervertebral discs (especially the one between the last vertebra and the sacrum) and on the muscles of the lower back (*erector spinae* or *quadratus lumborum*). These forces may tear the muscles or force the disc to extrude—both extremely painful outcomes.

Consider the Olympic and power-lifting movements (the "clean" and the "deadlift"), wherein very heavy weights are lifted. These movements take advantage of the body's great strength when used efficiently—that is, when forces applied to it are distributed as widely as possible. This can occur only when all parts of the body involved in the movement can share the load—and this can occur only when the body is held in a particular configuration. In the trash can movement described, this is far from the case. The lessons to be learned from this are simple. When picking anything up, the following rules must be observed:

- Directly face the object to be lifted;

- Bend the knees and minimize bending forwards from the hips;

- Hold the trunk as straight as you can with a slight backwards arch in the lumbar spine (if you cannot maintain this shape while lifting, the weight is *too heavy* for you to lift);

- Have your weight evenly distributed through both hands and over both feet;

- Hold the object as close to the body as you can;

- Hold the object with straight arms, as far as practicable; and

- Take in a breath and hold it when performing the actual lifting movement.

Always focus your attention on what you are doing. This may seem like gratuitous advice, but most injuries occur when you are doing something physical while your attention is focused elsewhere. Never combine a lifting and twisting movement. These remarks apply to the typical untrained individual. Obviously, a discus thrower or similar athlete can ignore this advice, because he or she has trained hard to be able to do just this movement. However, unless you are such a specialist athlete, you would be well advised to observe these rules. Olympic and power lifters handle enormous weights in their events. If you observe them carefully, you will see that they obey all of these rules, *without exception*. Perhaps surprisingly, back injuries are rarer in these sports than in most other track and field events, despite the huge stresses they impose on the lower back.

The daily six

If you decide to do a few exercises from chapter one on a daily basis (the "limbering" approach described in *Planning a stretching routine*) here are my suggestions for routines, assuming you have recovered, and depending on the site of your problem.

For low back pain

Exercises 1 and 2 (treat this as one exercise), exercise 31, exercise 3, exercise 29 , exercise 5 and exercise 6 to finish.

For middle back pain

Exercises 1 and 2 (again, treat this pair as one exercise), exercise 12, exercise 14, exercise 3, exercise 28 and exercise 13 to finish.

For upper back and neck pain

Exercise 15, exercise 14, exercise 16, exercise 18, exercise 21 and exercise 3 to finish.

For whole-body suppleness

Exercises 1 and 2 (treat this as one exercise), exercise 29, exercise 6, exercise 14, exercise 31 and exercise 3 to finish.

Pointers to chapter four, causes, and chapter five, relaxation techniques

Chapter four deals with the causes of neck and back pain, and is a little more technical than preceding chapters. Chapter five deals with a simple approach to learning how to relax. A great deal has been written on this subject, and the consensus of opinion is that, especially with neck and back pain, the development of relaxation habits (which can be learned quite easily) speeds up the healing process. Applying these lessons will be the more difficult matter, but the motivation that has carried you this far should help you prevail. If you wish, you may proceed to chapter five, and return to chapter four at a later time.

THE CAUSES OF NECK AND BACK PAIN

This chapter gives an overview of the causes of back pain, from a number of different perspectives. Central to these explanations is the notion of cause, and this concept is used as an organizing theme for this section. The chapter also explores some of the reasons why the very idea of cause can be a problem with respect to common illnesses like neck and back pain. I discuss the workshops we have been conducting around Australia, and present the results of testing around 1,500 people. In this section, I expand upon the idea of pelvic obliquity as a cause, the nature of entrapment phenomena such as *piriformis syndrome* and Thoracic Outlet Compression Syndrome (TOCS), and an analysis of the significance of patterns of muscle imbalance is presented.

Why do we suffer back pain?

Looking at the illustration overleaf, we can see that the spine comprises 24 bones (seven cervical, twelve thoracic, and five, sometimes six, lumbar vertebrae) plus the five fused bones of the sacrum and the four fused bones of the coccyx, the tail bone. Each vertebra has a large, solid section, the *vertebral body*, and the intervertebral disc (the area indicated by diagonal lines) sits in between adjacent vertebral bodies, and is strongly bonded to them. The outer part of this tough, fibro-cartilage disc is the *annulus*; the central part is a soft core, the *nucleus*. The spinal cord passes through a bony ring, behind the disc; the extensions rearwards off this ring are the bones that form the articular surfaces of the spine, the *facet joints,* and the *processes,* the attachment points for the muscles. The cer-ical vertebrae have a rearwards-facing concavity, the thoracic vertebrae have a much larger radius rearwards-pointing convex curve, and the lumbar vertebrae have a concavity rearwards. Looking at the left-hand part of the illustration, we see that extensions of the spinal cord, the *segmental nerves*, exit the sheath of the spinal cord on both sides at all vertebral junctions. The nerves exiting the cervical vertebrae innervate the skin and muscles of the head and arm, the thoracic vertebrae's nerves innervate the internal organs and the muscles and skin of the trunk, and the lumbar and sacral nerves innervate the hips and legs.

There are many theories that try to explain why humans seem to be predisposed to neck and back pain. One leading anatomist claims that the lumbar lordosis (the curve of lumbar spine) is a major weakness of the body, due in part to the shearing forces present at the lumbosacral junction (that is, the joint between the fifth lumbar vertebra and the first sacral vertebra, L5–S1), and the evidence to support this is that most back operations are performed at this junction. Looking at the illustration overleaf and comparing it with the illustration accompanying exercise 33, we can see that this shear force will be increased as the curves of the spine are increased. This happens when the pelvis tilts forwards—an accompaniment to gaining too much weight, for example, or when the hip flexors become tighter, as might be the case if a great deal of time is spent sitting or driving.

Kapandji hypothesizes that this potential weakness arose from the transition from quadrupedal to bipedal (four-legged to two-legged) movement in our distant past. The human spine, which was originally a single curve anteriorly when our forebears moved around on all fours, became straight and then the lower part curved further backward to form the spine's present shape. According to some researchers, the normal lumbar lordosis is said to have resulted because the pelvis has not yet tilted far enough posteriorly during evolution. The same changes in curvature of the spine from

One theory of back weakness

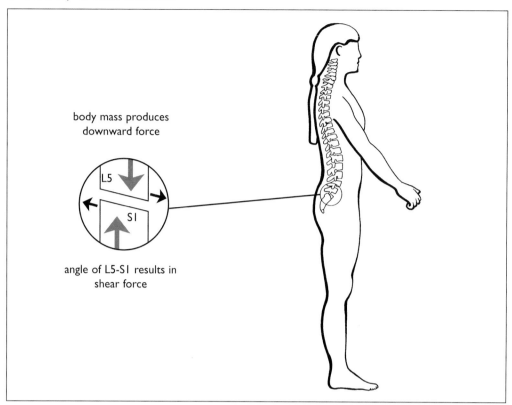

body mass produces
downward force

L5

S1

angle of L5-S1 results in
shear force

The three curves of the spinal column act as a shock absorber

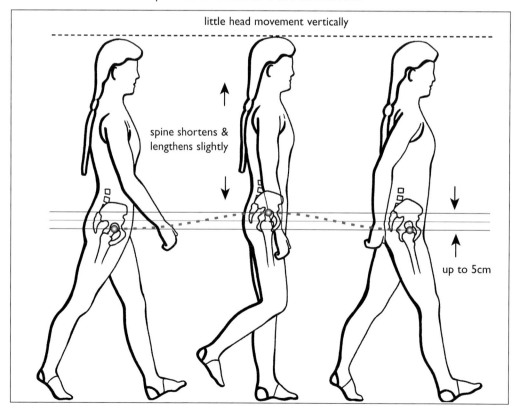

little head movement vertically

spine shortens &
lengthens slightly

up to 5cm

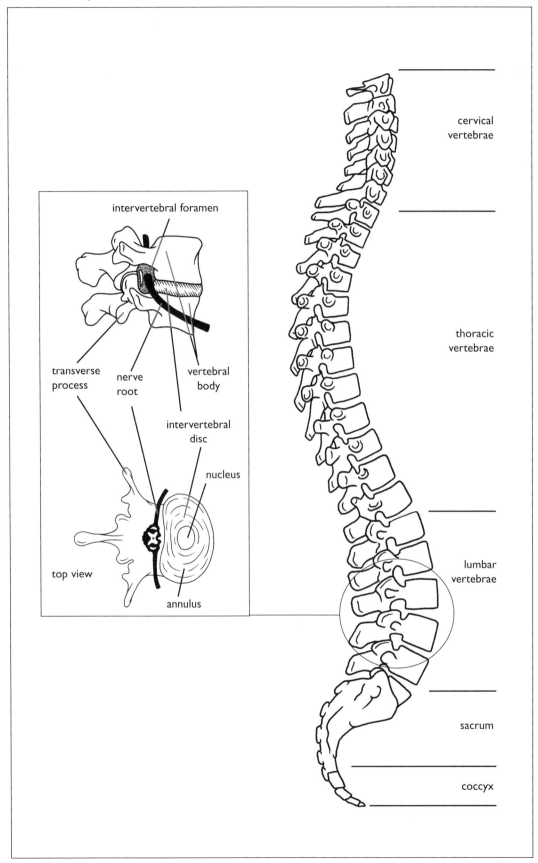

intervertebral foramen

transverse
process

nerve
root

vertebral
body

intervertebral
disc

nucleus

top view

annulus

cervical
vertebrae

thoracic
vertebrae

lumbar
vertebrae

sacrum

coccyx

anterior to posterior are observed during the first ten years of life; thus "the phylogenic [evolutionary] changes are recapitulated during ontogeny [personal development]" (Kapandji, 1974, vol. III, p. 16). Henderson states that the lumbar spine of most quadrupedal vertebrates is a smooth anterior curve. Animals with a lordotic curve—such as dogs and horses—also suffer spinal problems. Thus, humans are "predisposed to [certain kinds of] low back pathology" (1985, p. 1156). An increasing number of chiropractors specialize in treating horses and dogs for back problems.

However, there are also convincing arguments for a contrary position. Examination of the variation in vertebral structure from the skull to the pelvis has shown that the articular processes (the parts of the vertebrae that resist the shear forces mentioned above) are more widely separated at L_5, and the vertebral body itself wedge-shaped (as seen from the side) to help resist this tendency. It is also true that a condition called *spondylo-olisthesis* (or commonly abbreviated to spondylolisthesis) exists, where part of the bony support structure of the spine is fractured. This may be seen on radiographic analysis (X-ray), and frequently is asymptomatic. From the larger context, the shape of the spine can also be seen as a superb adaptation mechanism—without its three curves (see the illustration on the previous page for details) the spine would have almost no longitudinal shock-absorbing protection, and every step would jar the skull. Film analysis has shown that when a person is walking or running the head hardly moves at all vertically, and most of the vertical pelvic movement is absorbed by the curves of the spine tightening and releasing slightly. Moreover, engineering analyses have shown that the curves of the spine significantly increase its resistance to axial compression loads, in comparison to a straight spine (Kapandji, vol. III, p. 20 ff.). Another way of looking at the spine is to see it as a physical solution to the multiple objectives of how to design a structure with minimum weight, maximum strength and mobility, and which can move efficiently in an environment of gravity.

The argument of maladaptive evolutionary change does not explain why some people never suffer back pain. The arguments for and against humans being prone to back problems because of basic "design" faults are equally convincing—or unconvincing. No overwhelmingly persuasive evidence exists for either position. The pragmatic position taken here is, "this is how we are," and that the arguments are of more interest to anatomists than those who wish to do something about the problem. In an important sense the arguments are limiting: what we are trying to determine is what can we do to help the problem—if we did believe that there is a basic weakness in the structure, our resolve to do something about it would be compromised.

Nonetheless, the vertebral column has long been accepted by most doctors as the cause in the great majority of episodes of chronic back pain. As Ganora states "there is little doubt that most cases are due to derangement of the intervertebral joint in association with 'degeneration' of the disc and arthrosis of the facet joints." In the following sentence he says "Exactly which structures within this motion segment are the actual sources of pain remains conjectural" (Ganora, 1984, p. 55). Schwarzer claims that "more than 95% of patients with low back pain suffer from mechanical back pain" (1996, p. 108). Other researchers take a different view. Murtagh says that "most back pain is minor, caused by ligamentous and muscular strains which usually subside without treatment; the general practitioner sees the more severe cases" (1983, p. 322). He states in his survey of 1,000 patients that "spinal derangement" accounted for over 67% of back pain. Expert opinion is divided over whether disc protrusion or "overriding" of the pain-sensitive apophyseal joints [or facet joints] is the cause (Murtagh, 1983). Schwarzer argues that, because the intervertebral disc itself is richly supplied with nerves, they are a potential source of pain, and in his guide to physicians he lists the intervertebral disc as the most likely cause of pain. He distinguishes between "discogenic" pain and nerve root pain, the former being pain arising from the disc itself, and the latter characterised by referred pain in the hip or leg (Schwarzer, 1996).

The disc has long been a focus of medicine in respect of neck and back pain. Fifty years ago, a paper published by Mixter and Barr provided the theoretical foundation and justification for a wave of back operations over the next two decades, described by one commentator as "the dynasty of the disc" (Henderson, 1985). This early paper first used the term "intervertebral disc lesion," often called a "slipped disc" disc in common usage. The term refers to the partial or complete extrusion of the soft, gelatinous center (*nucleus*) of the intervertebral disc through the tough outer part of the disc, the *annulus*. Other terms used are "bulging" (when the extrusion is incomplete, but where deformation of the shape of the disc can be determined), or "prolapsed," where the material has extruded beyond the normal border of the disc. One kind of disc prolapse is illustrated on page 162.

During the 1940s and 1950s, many exploratory laminectomies (operations that partly or completely excise disc material) were performed with indifferent results (Henderson, 1985), illustrating a connection between theory and practice. One researcher claimed that this "mammoth surgical exercise" was inevitable, because the solution appeared simple—removal of the disc (or part of the disc) would cure the problem (Taylor, cited by Twomey, 1974). As is now well accepted, this was not the case. However, even today the accepted wisdom at the first point of contact most patients have with the medical profession—the general practitioner—is that some kind of disc or vertebral joint problem is the most likely cause of acute or chronic back pain.

However, radiography reveals degenerative change in the vertebral structures of most people over 30 years old, and about one fifth of this population never suffers back pain (Laughlin, 1989). Epidemiological studies suggest that about half of the patients suffering acute back pain at any time are well within a week and over 85% are well within a month. As far as we know, vertebral pathology does not change significantly within these time frames. Further confusing the issues are the results of a study published in the New England Journal of Medicine (Jensen *et al.*, 1994). Using MRI (Magnetic Resonance Imaging) technology, the researchers found that two-thirds of a group studied had the sort of abnormalities or disease which would be judged as the cause of pain had these been found in a back pain sufferer—yet the group had been selected from a sample of people who had never had back pain. The inconsistency in these results may be explained by suggesting that pathology exists benignly until other factors make it significant. However, because of medicine's desire to establish causal chains, diagnostic procedures designed to reveal the presence of pathology are employed. If pathology is found, back pain will be attributed to it (Laughlin, 1989). This interpretation has received a great deal of support in recent times (see, for example, Loeser, 1996; Vernon, 1996). The diagnostic dilemma is even more complicated if sciatica is present because most practitioners regard it as evidence of segmental nerve impingement, yet as I will show below, there is at least one muscular cause of the same symptoms.

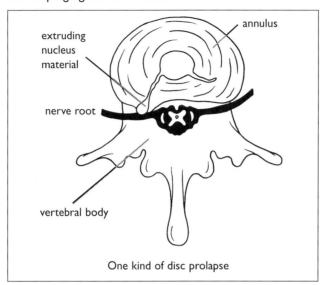

Posterolateral (back-side) extrusion of intervertebral disc impinging on nerve root

annulus

extruding nucleus material

nerve root

vertebral body

One kind of disc prolapse

Chiropractic and osteopathy

A great many people do not go to a doctor if they have neck or back problems, but seek the assistance of a chiropractor or an osteopath. Chiropractic and osteopathy both rely on a particular "lesion" of the spine as the main cause of back pain. They use the term *subluxation*, which is defined as "a clinically significant disturbance of joint movement or position which responds to manipulation" (Charlton, 1988). The Macquarie Dictionary describes a subluxation as a "partial dislocation" (Macquarie, 1981). Treatment consists of "long leverage mobilization techniques" (osteopaths) or "short leverage dynamic thrust techniques" (chiropractors), which are said to restore normal function to the joint in question (Bolton, 1987). Generally, the ministrations of osteopaths are said to be more gentle than those of chiropractors, and involve a preparatory massage of the area to be manipulated and greater attention is paid to the possible soft tissue causes of the subluxation. However, the differences between the two practices is dwindling and cross-fertilization of techniques is common and increasing. One chiropractor (trained in the U.S. and holding postgraduate qualifications) recently told me that he considered the differences between the practice of different chiropractors at least as significant as the alleged differences between the two professions, and that there is an increasing focus on soft-tissue problems.

It is perhaps of some concern that the subluxation both professions rely on has never been "proved" as an "independently verifiable, clinically significant entity" (Charlton, 1988). It needs to be said here that "proved," in this context, means proved to the satisfaction of the western medical profession, which attempts to understand illness in terms of cause and process. If one adopts the empirical perspective, ignores process, and simply considers the relation between problem, intervention and outcome (in other words, treating the intervention techniques as a "black box"), it is clear that significant changes are brought about to a patient's condition by manipulation. Chiropractors and osteopaths themselves have no problem with the concept in either theory or practice, nor do most of their large number of patients. This finding may have more to do with the standards of evidence being applied to the problem than any shortcomings in the techniques—that is, it may be the case that the standards of proof being sought are unreasonably restrictive. There is little doubt that many people gain relief from their problems through chiropractic and osteopathic techniques. Western medicine itself has a long history of using manipulation, sometimes performed under anesthetic (Maitland, 1986).

Oriental medicine

Various forms of oriental medicine are also used to treat back pain. The approach is based on an understanding of the body that differs significantly from that of western scientific medicine, chiropractic and osteopathy. The two latter treatments have allied themselves with western medicine in Australia only quite recently, following a pattern of discrimination similar to that seen in both the United States and Great Britain in earlier times. In contrast to the biological–physical (biophysical) approach of western medicine, oriental medicine is based on a distinctly different cosmology. The oriental systems postulate a flow of energy (*ch'i,* in Chinese, or *ki,* in Japanese) around the body through fourteen channels called meridians—lines of energy which flow around the body connecting the familiar acupuncture points. Disruptions to the normal flow of energy are considered to be the cause of disease (including illnesses like back pain), and accordingly an approach aimed at rebalancing this flow is used to help the problem. Treatment uses manual pressure (*shiatsu,* or *acupressure*), needles (*acupuncture*), heat applied to the acupuncture points judged to be effective in restoring this balance (*moxibustion*), or herbs prescribed to affect particular internal organs. Interestingly, it is common that such practitioners are as likely to treat areas far removed from the site of the patient's complaint as the area itself. In cases of back pain, the determination of the cause of the problem is normally made with reference to disturbances to meridians and their associated organ systems rather than to the structures of the back itself. The oriental systems can also avail themselves of various exercise forms. However, in contrast to physiotherapy or the like, the exercise is not explicitly designed to stretch or strengthen the muscles involved. Practitioners of oriental medicine usually claim that the purpose of the exercise is to restore a desirable or harmonious energy flow.

Acute pain

Western medicine is at its best treating the sort of back pain that results from acute trauma, such as a car accident. Acute trauma (for example, a compression injury that might crush particular vertebrae or their discs) can be extremely dangerous, with a risk of partial or complete paralysis if left untreated. Such paralysis is generally caused by mechanical derangement of the spinal cord or compression of segmental nerves, which exit from the spinal column between pairs of vertebrae. (This condition is often referred to as "nerve impingement.") Surgery is used to relieve the pressure on the nerves, and sometimes bone grafts are used to stabilize the pairs of vertebrae involved if the damage to the vertebrae is severe.

The site of the injury can be inferred from the location of what are called "neurological deficits." This term refers to patterns of loss of sensation, tingling in the muscles of the legs or feet, or loss of movement in specific muscle groups. Maps of the body called *dermatome* ("skin") and *myotome* ("muscle") charts show the relationships between particular areas of the skin or specific muscles, and their innervating nerves. These charts are used to identify the involved nerve and to infer the site of the damage. MRI or CAT (Computerized Axial Tomography; sometimes abbreviated to "CT") scans are used at the site (and usually a segment or two above and below) to more precisely identify both the site and nature of the lesion. However, this kind of acute segmental nerve impingement probably accounts for less than 5% of cases of acute back pain on the current figures. The most important question to answer is whether neurological signs exist—if they do, seek the assistance of your family doctor, to rule out the possibility of these sorts of problems.

Another common cause of neck or back pain is associated with acute muscle spasm. If the spasm is located in the neck muscles, the condition is known as *torticollis* (Latin for "twisted neck") or perhaps more familiarly, a "wry" neck. Muscle spasm is a strong, involuntary muscular contraction that you are unable to relax. The cause of such a condition is sometimes unclear—it may be the precursor to a cold or a bout of the flu, sleeping near an open window, or the result of unaccustomed activity. If the latter, the condition probably results from very small-scale lesions ("microtrauma" or small ruptures) to the muscle fibers themselves, causing a vigorous contraction of the surrounding fibers that may be an involuntary protective mechanism to prevent further injury.

If a similar microtrauma is responsible for an episode of acute back pain (particularly likely if you suspect that unaccustomed activity is the cause), take heart in the statistics. No matter how agonizing in the first instance (and this kind of pain can be so severe that some people cannot get out of bed), more than half such patients are better within a week, and more than 85% recover completely within three weeks. The best figures available suggest that after two to three months, fewer than 3% have any ongoing problems. Most general practitioners used to advise bed rest for a few days with appropriate NSAIDs (nonsteroidal antiinflammatory drugs, like aspirin), but active rest is now the more common recommendation. This usually involves avoiding the activity judged to be primarily responsible, and often includes advice to seek physiotherapy or massage. Much less common are problems like *ankylosing spondylitis,* a rheumatic disorder (20 per 1,000 cases presented); less frequent causes of acute pain are internal problems such as a urinary tract or kidney infection, or malignancy (the last mentioned cause found in 0.3 per 1,000; Schwarzer, 1996). Occasionally, muscle spasm results from disc prolapse (and which can be accompanied by sciatica) or from partial or complete fractures of the vertebrae (more common in women, particularly postmenopausal). Further consideration of other possible causes of sciatica is made later in this chapter.

Chronic pain

It is commonly accepted that most people will suffer back pain on some occasion in life. The main reason that people regard back pain so seriously is that when it occurs it is completely debilitating. A pulled muscle in the arm or leg is certainly inconvenient, and perhaps even painful, but many of life's normal activities can continue until the injury heals. As anyone who has suffered can attest, this is not the case with back pain—one's whole life, in its smallest and largest parts, is affected.

How much worse, then, is the plight of the sufferer of chronic neck or back pain? All aspects of life are affected to some degree—work, relationships, and recreational activities. The main focus of this book is chronic pain, or recurring pain and its alleviation. Before considering possible predisposing factors, one important question to be answered is whether your chronic pain continues unremittingly through the night. If this is the case, discuss the condition with your doctor to eliminate possible malignancies. Malignancy is the cause of back pain in about 1% of patients (Murtagh, 1985, although compare with Schwarzer's much lower figures, above).

Loss of disc height is commonly offered as an explanation for chronic back pain. The theory is that, as "normal" wear and tear to the intervertebral discs occurs, the discs lose some of their thickness. In fact, everyone loses about half an inch in height from morning to evening daily, as water is lost from all discs due to the compression force on the structures (the effect of gravity on the body's mass), and regained when we sleep. As mentioned previously, the segmental nerves exit the spine from the spinal cord through a space created by pairs of notches in adjoining vertebrae, not through fixed "holes." In the normal individual, there is enough space between the various structures—including the disc, a number of ligaments, and the *dura mater,* the sheath of the spinal cord through which the nerve must exit—for normal bending of the spine in any of its directions to have no compression effects on the nerves.

However, these spaces become narrower as disc height is lost. If enough disc thickness is lost, the surrounding structures can apply pressure to the segmental nerves, causing pain at the site of the pressure, and sometimes pain at more distant locations (*radicular,* or referred pain). Reduced disc thickness may also result in increased pressure on the facet joints, the sliding joints of the vertebrae, which are rich in nerves. Loss of disc height can also cause familiar *sciatica* (literally, pain in the sciatic nerve). Although this explanation may account for the primary cause in the extreme case, it is unlikely to be the whole explanation. Even sufferers of chronic back pain have good days, with little or no pain; accordingly, it seems likely that other factors besides vertebral pathology must also play a causal role.

Muscle tension as cause

The expression "muscle tension" is often used imprecisely, and with a negative connotation—but a certain degree of tension is required in the muscles for maintenance of posture, the same tension creates sufficient pressure in the veins to return the blood to the heart, and so on. This slight, continuous healthy tension is called *tonus.* The sort of tension that most people mean when they use the term is elevated tonus, or muscle tension increased beyond that required for the standard functions, and if sufficiently elevated, will signal discomfort initially, and if it continues, pain. There are many causes of this kind of tension, including the stress of daily life.

One contributing cause of neck and back pain can be tension (henceforth, we shall be using "tension" to mean elevated tonus) held in the muscles surrounding the site of an earlier injury. Tension increases in muscles surrounding any kind of physical trauma. It is thought to be a protective mechanism, to limit further injury to an area by limiting its movement (technically referred to as "splinting" or "bracing"). We become aware of this tension by the sensations of reduced movement in the part concerned, and the sensation of pain as the limit of this reduced movement is reached. If the tension is held for a long time (from weeks to years) a number of effects are noticed. One is that the protective tension, rather than serving a useful limiting function of brief duration, becomes a habit. A "feedback loop" is set up between the muscle fibers and the central nervous system, so that the pain signals cause a restimulation of the contracting fibers. If this continues, it may be accompanied by systemic changes to the relationship between the nerves and the muscle fibers, until (to continue the computer metaphors) the pain–contraction condition becomes "hard-wired" into the system: in addition to the pain signals, proprioceptive signals are interpreted as pain in a process called "sensitization." Damasio has found that an area in the brain called the *somatosensory cortex* contains a representation of all patterns of tension held in the muscles of the body. One's "postural signature" is "recorded" here. If, for any reason, one's way of holding or using the body is altered for some length of time, the somatosensory cortex changes to reflect this new "normal" (Damasio, 1995). Whether this new norm is desirable (from an independent perspective) is another matter. Such long-held tension in muscles can lead to changes at the cellular level, and collagen (a "string"-like protein) may be deposited in the area, forming hard knots in the affected muscles. The resulting changes are known by various names like fibrosis. If this condition is left untreated, the condition can become very difficult to change.

Following any injury where muscle cells are ruptured (where bruising occurs), collagen fibers are initially laid down at random. Electron microscope photographs show that the resulting fibers run in all directions initially. Over time, the fibers align themselves in response to forces applied to them. The crucial lesson is that knots in muscles following injury, or the often dramatic reduction in range of movement often observed after trauma, can result from healing itself. If the new collagen is not stressed in a way that mimics the demands of normal life, the affected muscle will have a reduced range of movement. Stress drives adaptation. For this reason, to restore normal function it is essential to stretch an injured part (very carefully, initially) and then strengthen it.

Another possible effect, without any detectable physiological change in the tissues involved, is that a particular pattern or way of holding the body may result—an altered postural signature. Such a pattern may be as difficult to change as a more physiologically based change. For example, consider someone who has had a broken leg set, and wears a plaster for six weeks or so. When the plaster is removed and physiotherapy has reestablished the previous size, strength and tone of the leg, a patient may still walk in a way that favors the leg. This altered movement pattern can persist for months or even years and can be extremely difficult to alter.

Emotional factors also play a role in chronic neck or back pain. The distinction between the physical and the mental becomes less clear the closer one looks at the way the whole body works, and Damasio's excellent book *Descartes' Error* explores the complex mechanisms involved. Nonetheless, the distinction can be useful, providing one realizes that it is one made for our convenience. Emotional factors refer to a range of attitudes and behaviors, from a more-or-less conscious choice to remove oneself from an undesirable situation by becoming ill (hence legitimating the absence) to normal reactions to stress or fatigue. Although not as directly obvious a cause as a trauma, the effects may well be as debilitating, and you must consider these factors in your treatment.

The great psychotherapist Wilhelm Reich coined the term "character armor" to describe the tendency of the injured child to accrete protective layers that, if left untreated, become the protective armor experienced (and displayed) by the adult. By armor, he referred to the great range of emotional or behavioral problems afflicting adults, and which always have physical correlates in patterns of held tension. Such armor has the well-known advantage of protection, but at the cost of rigidity and pain. He concluded that trauma experienced by the psyche manifests itself at the physical level of experience as tightness in the muscles, organ dysfunction, and pain. One of his solutions was a form of massage. Central to his approach to curing a patient's problem was restoration of normal physical function. Reich believed that returning the body's function to normal also healed the original injury to the psyche—"stored" in the tissues of the body—so that the complaint did not return. Reich's seminal work must be considered the genesis of the many "body work" schools around us today—over 200 distinct approaches, according to a recent count.

Other factors contributing to neck and back pain

Based on my experience, most people assume that they are symmetrical, but this is rarely the case. *Structural* asymmetry is common. A number of studies have examined the prevalence of leg-length inequality in the general population. The authors of a review of six studies concluded that "about 7% (range 4–8%) of the adult population with no history of low back pain have lower limb inequality of 1 cm [just under half an inch] or more" (Giles and Taylor, 1985). Other studies have found a significant correlation between low back pain and leg-length inequality (see, for example, Friberg, 1983; Matheson *et al.,* 1987); and other researchers have found no significant correlation (see, for example, Grundy & Roberts, 1984; Soukka *et al.,* 1991). The studies cited have considered radiographs (some used whole-body scans; others measured between landmarks such as *greater trochanter,* the palpable bone of the leg near the hip joint, and *lateral malleolus,* the outside ankle bone). Many factors may confound such measurements, and will be discussed below. Additionally, these assessments do not consider the muscular dimension, either in terms of development or function (comparisons of strength and flexibility). Ordinarily, muscles are invisible to the technologies used to see inside the body, including X-rays, MRIs and CAT scans.

Assuming that leg-length difference plays a causal role in back pain (and perhaps neck pain too), it would be expected that the proportion of people suffering neck or back pain who display this difference would be greater than in the general population. In my clinic, about 75% of patients with chronic back pain have a significant difference in leg length. The difference is significant if determinable by the tests described in chapter one—if there is no apparent difference, it may be that there is no difference or that the difference is one which the body can cope with without too many problems. The conclusion of leg-length difference is reached only when a sufficient number of the indicators mentioned coincide. This proportion is much higher than that reported in other studies (for example, Giles and Taylor, 1985, who state 18.3% and Rock, 1988, who states 10.9%). Part of the apparent discrepancy in these figures is due to the nine-millimeter (just under seven-sixteenths of an inch) threshold chosen in the studies; that is, only patients with differences greater than this were considered to demonstrate leg-length inequality. For example, Rock's study found that a further 38.5% of the chronic sufferers had a leg-length difference of between five and nine millimeters (between three-sixteenths and seven-sixteenths of an inch). Recalculation using three-sixteenths of an inch as the threshold of significance yields figures of around 50% of the sample groups cited. One explanation for the much higher percentage of patients displaying leg-length inequality in my clinic may be that I am seeing a proportion of patients who have not responded to other approaches, and in whom leg-length difference is a causal factor.

Why the nine millimeter threshold was chosen in the early studies is not apparent from close reading of them. Differences as small as 3 to 5 millimeters may be significant in patients with narrow hips, or where certain aspects of lifestyle dominate the adaptive mechanisms. For example, if the nine-millimeter threshold is significant for a 185 cm male, a lesser difference will produce an identical tilting of the pelvis of a 150 cm male (as measured in degrees from horizontal) if his

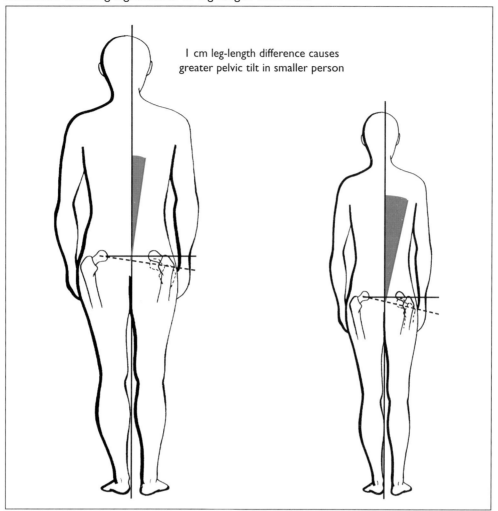

I cm leg-length difference causes greater pelvic tilt in smaller person

hips are narrower than the taller person's (see the illustration). For an extreme example of predisposing lifestyle factors, consider one of my patients, a world-class triathlete. Very careful independent assessment of his skeletal structure suggests a horizontal tilting of the pelvis of only 2 to 3 millimeters, yet he displayed dramatic asymmetrical muscular development in the lumbar and thoracic areas of the sort described below, and a pronounced asymmetry of function consistent with the structural asymmetry. He also runs 100 miles per week in the volume phases of his training. As the triathlon is one of the most symmetrical of activities, we concluded that his asymmetry was his body's attempt to adapt his structure to this load.

Accordingly, structural asymmetry of this sort may or may not have consequences—it depends on two questions: where it exists, and at which point it becomes significant. Any factor that disturbs the balance of the body *may* be significant, as we live in a world pervaded by gravity. For this reason, leg-length inequality is more likely to be significant than arm-length inequality, because the legs bear our weight. At which point such inequality is likely to become significant will be explored below, but this question depends crucially on lifestyle: an inequality that would be insignificant for a normal, relatively sedentary person could be highly significant for an athlete whose sport is played in the vertical, load-bearing position, or someone whose work is done mainly in the standing position. As discussed in chapter one, we consider visible or palpable right/left differences in the development of the lumbar and thoracic extensor muscles to be evidence of one kind, and asymmetric patterns of flexibility to be evidence of another kind, assuming relatively symmetrical activities in the patient's lifestyle.

Other structural problems may be seen by looking at the body from the side. For example, there may be an exaggerated curve of the upper spine (*kyphosis*), or of the lower back (*lordosis*). Kyphosis is always accompanied by an exaggerated extension of the neck (a backwards arching), necessary to hold the head level. This structural condition alone can produce strong tension in the muscles needed to hold the head in this position. It is safe to say that any deviation from a posited "ideal" will require some compensatory adaptation from another part. It is generally accepted in engineering theory that the maximum strength of any symmetrical structure is achieved by the widest distribution of forces throughout the whole structure; this avoids stress concentrations. Patients with a structural problem always have increased tension in particular muscles—those required to do extra work to support the body's shape. These tighter areas almost always coincide with the loci of pain.

Asymmetry in the balances between flexibility and strength in various areas around the body can also produce deviations in the ideal shape of the spine. It is useful sometimes to consider strength as a lack of flexibility—or to consider flexibility as being equivalent to insufficient strength—due to the relationship of these properties in forming the characteristic shape of the individual. For example, tight *psoas* and *iliacus* muscles (*iliopsoas*, the hip flexors) together can tilt the pelvis forwards, producing the familiar lumbar lordosis (sway back). This does not involve structural asymmetry or spinal abnormality. In such cases, the excessive tension (strength) of these muscles is not balanced by an appropriate group, such as the abdominal muscles. Another way to consider the same problem is to assert that the iliopsoas muscles are insufficiently flexible. The reasons for making this distinction will become clearer when we see how the two conceptualizations offer two different solutions. Before exploring this idea further, let us explore the notion of posture, from a structural and functional perspective, which will add meaning to the standard aesthetic dimension of this idea.

What is good posture?

Good posture is not a form imposed on our own structure, as an externally applied ideal. Some bodywork schools attempt to impose an ideal of posture by creating good postural habits. In this approach, the individual consciously imposes certain ways of moving or holding the body. The approach relies on repeating these self-instructions until they become one's own ways of moving and holding the body. However, the imposition of mental models alone is generally not a very efficient way to alter the basic structure and function of one's body. Continual imposition of these models can result in a somewhat mechanical or "robotic" way of moving that works against the spontaneity of good movement. Until the models themselves have "become" you, you tend to forget the ideal form when you are distracted or fatigued. Good posture should be effortless and involuntary—most babies and animals have perfect posture. The path to gracefulness and ease of movement does not need additional constraints. This is not to deny that the many hours of repetition of movements done by dancers and gymnasts (not to mention yoga teachers and the like) help to make them graceful in ordinary life. But unless you have these goals foremost in your life, it is inefficient to use these approaches to gain ease of movement and good posture.

A better approach for most people is to apply certain kinds of stress to the body so that the body itself changes. Sufficient change yields good posture and graceful movement. The spinoffs are a reduction in pain and a feeling of physical freedom. In contrast to animals and babies, adults can pursue these goals efficiently, by analyzing their own form and applying corrective techniques. The most significant differences between adults and babies or animals are self-awareness and knowledge, and these faculties can be used to improve posture and ease of movement.

According to physiotherapists (Kendall *et al.*, 1971, p. 19) good posture may be determined using a plumb line. If the body is viewed from the side, and if the weight of the plumb line is placed a little forward of one ankle bone (*external malleolus*), the line attached to the weight will pass slightly forward of the axis of the knee joint and slightly behind the axis of the hip joint. The line will be parallel with a number of lumbar vertebrae, run through the shoulder joint, and align with the back of the ear. Examine the illustration. From the side the body is not by any means straight, and the curves of the spine are clearly seen. In this plane (the *sagittal* plane) the shape of the spine can be seen as the solution to a number of conflicting needs—to absorb shock (especially from running or walking), to protect the spinal cord, and to use the minimum amount of energy to maintain its shape.

Notice that there is no symmetry in this plane. The front half (that section forward of the line) bears no relation in terms of shape to the back half. However, if a person with good posture is standing in a relaxed fashion, about half of the body's weight will be on either side of this line. The center of gravity in the average person is slightly in front of the first or second sacral segment (recall that the sacrum is the lowest, fused part of the spine). This suggests that the center of gravity roughly coincides with the hip joint. In contrast, from behind the symmetry of the body is clear—a right and a left half. good posture is regarded as having the ankles in a stable configuration, neither rolling in nor out. The Achilles tendon should be straight from the heel to the calf muscle. The legs should appear straight, with the hips level. The spine should be straight, with the shoulders level and the head held above the spine and in line with it. From the front, the knees should point straight ahead. The weight of the body should be carried evenly over both feet.

Ideal posture is simply that shape the body adopts as its "minimum-energy configuration"—the shape that requires the minimum amount of energy to support. Try this little experiment. Stand up and place the back of one hand across the small of your back. Lean your body very slightly forwards or backwards, until you find a point where the large

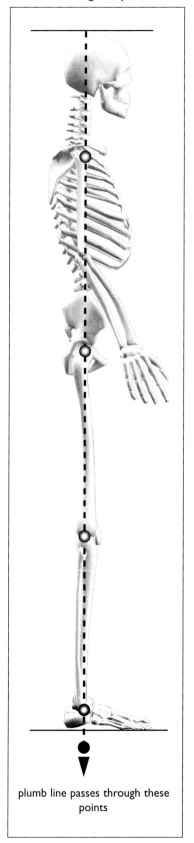

Schematic of good posture

plumb line passes through these points

170

muscles running up both sides of the spine are completely relaxed. Notice that these muscles are relaxed even though you are standing up and your body is supporting its weight. Ligaments, tendons and joints are providing the support. Now lean forwards from this position a small amount—less than an inch will produce the effect. Immediately, these long muscles tighten considerably—even though the weight of the body has not changed. By leaning forward though, the configuration of the body has changed, and hence the muscles are required to do extra work. From this example, you can see that if your posture is inefficient by even a small amount, you must do a considerable amount of extra work to support your body.

Assuming this idea of minimum-energy configuration is correct, your structure (the alignment of the body) or your available range of movement at particular joints may not permit you to realize this form. Your minimum-energy shape may in fact require quite an effort. To return to the theme of an earlier paragraph, there is not much point in trying to impose an ideal form on a less than ideal structure, conceptualized in these terms. Optimal results are gained by working at the structural level, working slowly to change the shape of the spine, its support mechanisms and, critically, the muscles that affect this shape.

Consider the body from the side view in more detail. With respect to neck pain, one needs to assess whether the curve of the thoracic spine is excessive. Recall the simple experiment. Although everyone's body is unique, if your head is carried sufficiently far in front of the shoulders, all the neck muscles involved in extension (that is, the muscles which bring the head backwards) will be contracted whenever you are in your normal vertical load-bearing position—even when you are sitting down. The main thing to look for is whether the curve of the thoracic spine is causing you to hold the head in front of that ideal posited position. If this is so, various muscles are doing work that is unnecessary in a better-balanced person, simply to hold your head level.

A similar analysis applies to the shape of the lumbar spine. Although excessive lumbar curve (lumbar lordosis, or "sway" back) is often cited as a cause of low back pain, this explanation may be a little simplistic. Sometimes, someone with well-developed buttocks can give the impression of a sway back to a casual inspection that mistakes the curve of the buttocks for the course of the spine. The shape of the whole spine needs to be considered. For example, many a dancer or gymnast gives the impression of having a sway back for the reason just given, but has a thoracic spine with an ideal gentle curve, and shoulders that sit squarely, and a head carried perfectly. This is not a true sway back. In addition, such athletes usually have very powerful abdominal muscles (which play an important support role for the spine in dynamic movement) so that even if (technically speaking) one of them does have a sway back, it may be well compensated and hence should not be considered a problem.

In some people, very tight lower back muscles can prevent the spine's normal reverse curve from straightening, let alone allowing it to bend forward. This, too, can give the impression of a sway back. Some people also have a more pronounced curve in the lumbar spine, but without any dysfunction, and with great mobility. To label such form as a sway back serves little purpose. Finally, just because there is no symmetry between the front and back halves of the body, the determination and assessment of "normal" in this plane remains problematic.

When one looks at the body from behind, asymmetry may be seen relatively easily. Perhaps of most importance with respect to neck and back pain is the height of the hips. To this point, we have discussed hip levelness in terms of leg-length inequality, but a number of other structural

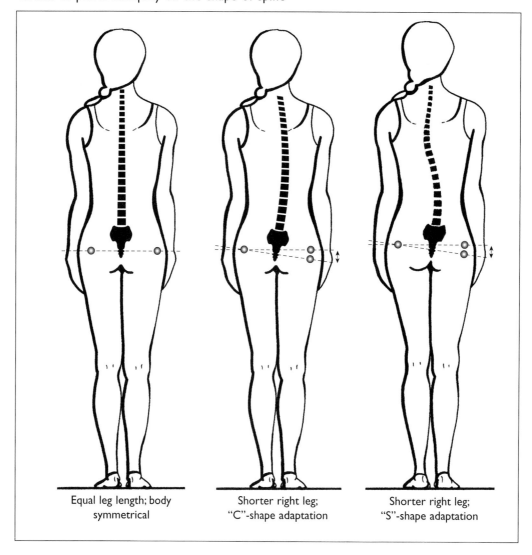

Equal leg length; body symmetrical

Shorter right leg; "C"-shape adaptation

Shorter right leg; "S"-shape adaptation

factors may produce the same result, and frequently these factors seem not to have been considered in research that has looked at this problem. If one ankle *pronates* (rolls inwards) excessively and the other is normal, the hip on the pronating ankle side will be lower. If a researcher measures between hip and outside ankle bone (a common technique) this factor will not show up, and the statistics will underestimate the extent of obliquity in individual subjects being measured, and will underestimate its frequency in the population studied. Similarly if the angles between the neck of the femur and the femur itself are not the same on both legs: measurement of the distance between the *greater trochanter* and the ankle bone (or floor) may indicate equal leg length, but the pelvis will tilt towards the side of the smaller angle. If a condition called *small hemipelvis* exists (where one half of the pelvis is significantly smaller than the other), the leg bones may well be identical and the person being tested still have one hip lower than the other; similarly for hip joints that are not located directly opposite one another in the pelvis. A person with any of these asymmetries

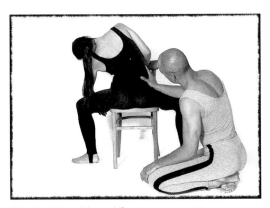

Hemipelvis and lateral flexion test position

may be recorded as having identical leg lengths in such studies, yet a visual inspection in the standing position may reveal a tilted pelvis.

If you suspect *small hemipelvis* may be related to your problem, ask someone to check the height of the hips from behind, while you are sitting with your hips on a table. The testing block may be used under each hip in turn, as in the leg-length test. The photograph shows the test position; additionally, Jennifer is leaning to one side to permit a comparison of lateral flexion, and if the lumbar area is visible the relative sizes of the lower back muscles will be visible. I suggest that this test be done if: i) the standing test indicates uneven hip bone heights, yet your partner tells you that the visible course of the spine appears straight, or ii) levelling the hips with a test block causes the spine to curve laterally, or iii) your recurring back pain occurs mainly while sitting (here, you may present a straight spine in the standing test, but will demonstrate an induced scoliosis when seated). Our recommendation for correction is a support for the smaller half of the pelvis to be used under that hip when seated. You may or may not require a leg-length correction.

All these factors have implications for the shape of the whole spine. Leaving aside questions of the effects of right–left arm dominance for a moment, if the right hip is actually lower than the left, then two adaptation patterns are commonly seen: either the three normal curves of the spine will be reproduced subtly in the plane running through both shoulders (the "S" shape shown in the illustration) or the spine will have a wider-radius "C"-shaped curve (the middle illustration). If the adaptation is "S"-shaped, the left shoulder will then be carried on the outside of a gently right-curving thoracic spine, as shown in the illustration, and may be carried higher than the right shoulder. If the adaptation is "C"-shaped, the right shoulder may well be carried higher. To the untrained eye, a difference in shoulder height may be difficult to see. It is often easier to appreciate by considering whether the fingers of one hand reach further down one leg than the other, assuming that the arms are the same length. Alternatively, if looking at the body from behind, the course of the spine may be more easily seen by inclining the body forward from the hips, as in the experiment mentioned above (the tightened muscles highlight the shape of the spine, especially if lit from the side).

Tests of leg-length inequality

Hip levelness (pelvic obliquity) is best tested in the standing position, as described in chapter one. The use of a support under each foot in turn will magnify any difference, as we have discussed. Here, I wish to argue for this approach versus the more common lying assessment techniques. In the conventional lying face-up (or face-down) approach to testing leg length, the practitioner holds the patient's heels (or feet) just off the bench, and applies an equal, gentle pull to both legs. The comparison is made by examining the heels, or lines drawn on the inside ankle bones. If one is closer to the practitioner, it is judged to be the longer leg. The problem with this test is that other factors may mask the difference completely, or even dominate it. In the extreme case the leg appearing as the longer one in this test may actually be shorter than its partner. For example, if the patient has occasioned trauma to *quadratus lumborum*, the oblique group of muscles, or the deep muscles of the lumbar spine (common in contact sports, for example), their contraction alone (in response to the trauma) will draw the hip on that side towards the ribs when the body is relaxed, or supported horizontally. This contraction can give the impression of the leg on the side of the injury being the shorter one, and the standing test described in chapter one may reveal the opposite. Leg length testing must be done in the standing position, because in the lying position, muscular contractions can pull the pelvis one way or another. It may be objected that the contracted muscles will disturb the alignment of the pelvis in the standing test, too. However, in the standing position with the body's weight firmly over both feet, it is the *body* that will be distorted—that is, the body alone will be drawn to the side of the injury. As we are concerned with the levelness of the hips in the first part of the test, this distortion can be ignored. If the contraction is extreme, however, assessment becomes difficult. One additional source of structural misalignment which may ramify to an apparent leg-length inequality is when the sacrum is tilted in relation to the pelvis. This condition should be visible using an appropriate X-ray technique and may be able to be corrected by manipulation. In such cases, I still recommend an analysis of the patient's structure and function as described, to try to determine the nature of the cause of this particular "adaptation," presuming that trauma is not the cause.

What effects can uneven hips have on the body?

Let us assume that you have found a leg-length difference and the difference seems to be about half an inch. How much correction should be used in the heel of the shoe? Before considering a specific amount, let us review the argument. My approach is partly based on the claim that a lateral curvature of the spine induced by a leg-length difference can cause back pain, most commonly through the uneven work done by the muscles of the laterally curved spine. In many people, this asymmetry is compensated by additional development of the muscles on the outside of the lumbar spine on the same side as the shorter leg and also on the opposite side to the shorter leg in the thoracic spine region, assuming an "S"-shaped adaptation, as shown in the illustration on page 172. This compensation provides two loci for pain, through two mechanisms. One is nerve impingement, and the other is simple muscular soreness brought about by particular muscles on one side of the spine having to do more work than on the other. This produces more

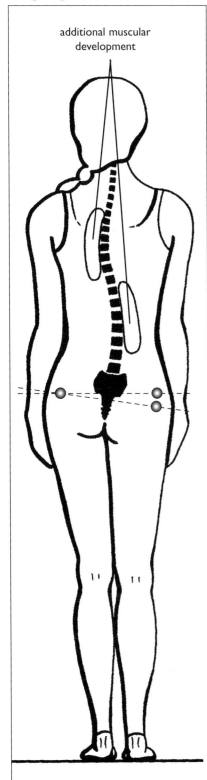

Simple model of possible effects of leg-length difference

additional muscular development

development in the affected muscles, but the muscles are tighter (normal state being more contracted than the muscles opposite) and they are closer to the fatigued state than the other side's weaker, though more relaxed, counterparts. This may explain in part the oft-reported tendency for episodes of back pain to follow periods of stress or fatigue—that is, the affected muscles reach their limit for doing work before the others.

However, these predictions of muscular development are not always borne out in practice, and (despite any predictive models to the contrary) you must try to find what factors are actually present. Other causes may confound the predictions I have outlined here. In such cases, deal with the functional or structural asymmetry you find. In persons displaying the "C"-shaped adaptation, the additional development is usually found on the outside of the entire curve, through the lumbar and thoracic regions. Perhaps contrary to expectations, in the majority of people we have tested, the better developed muscles (independent of the shape the spine has attained in adaptation) are *always* tighter on testing; that is, even though this additional development is found on the *outside* of the curve in question (and thus the back is already bending this way), a comparison of right and left lateral flexion reveals that bending in the direction of the existing curve—and hence stretching the better-developed muscles—is always more difficult than bending the other way. Stretching the larger muscles very often reproduces the problem pain.

Another related likely cause of *referred* pain is the nerve impingement mechanism mentioned above. That is, in daily life the *intervertebral foramina* (the pairs of notches through which the segmental nerves exit the spine) are narrower on the side of the longer leg, because the spine is tilted in this direction to distribute its load as evenly as possible and to achieve balance in all of life's activities. This adaptation is especially significant in upright load-bearing positions, and thus more likely to be causal in people who spend their life on their feet, or whose sport places similar demands on the skeleton. For confirming evidence, look at a worn pair of shoes. Generally, although not always, the sole of the shoe of the shorter leg is the more worn.

How thick should my heel lift be?

It will be clear from the discussion so far that the greater the leg-length difference, the greater its significance as a possible causal factor, even if other possible causes are present. A minor difference is unlikely to be significant, because it is within the body's capacity to adapt without negative consequences. Accordingly, the *first* fractions of any difference are more significant (with respect to the problem) than the last fractions. Addressing part of a larger difference is thus more likely to yield positive benefits than addressing a difference which is closer to the balanced position. For example, if one patient has a leg-length difference of three-quarters of an inch and another has a difference of three-eighths, inserting a lift of three-eighths of an inch into the shoe of the shorter leg will yield far more dramatic results in the patient with the larger difference. The reason is that back pain, like any other pain, is a phenomenon with a threshold. If stimulation is below the threshold, pain is not experienced, even though the cause of the stimulation may be present. The three-eighths insert causes the same change in angle of the pelvis with respect to the theoretical transverse plane in both cases (let us say a few degrees). However, the change is of greater significance in the patient with the larger leg-length difference because the lateral curvature of this patient's spine is closer to the threshold where capacity for work or impingement is reached.

For these reasons, an insert of between three-sixteenths and three-eighths of an inch should be used in most cases. A greater thickness is not recommended for three reasons. Assuming that the patient has adapted during life to this structural difference (even if the adaptation is incomplete or only partially effective), correcting the whole difference may render these adaptations maladaptive, and hence likely to cause other problems. The second reason is a practical one. Most shoe styles will accept an insert of this order of thickness without the discomfort of the heel not being securely held in the shoe. The third reason is one of economy. If a small correction yields the desired result, it is to be preferred. It is a basic tenet of physical medicine to use the smallest stimulation of the body's adaptive mechanisms which will serve the desired purpose, and is least likely to have undesirable side effects.

Is right- or left-handedness related to the problem?

In any population displaying these kinds of adaptations, various factors may mask the differences mentioned. One arm may be longer than the other, for example, confusing the visual assessment. You can check this by lying down with the shoulders resting on the floor and extending the arms up from the chest, with the fingers brought together over the center of the chest. Another person can check this for you. As mentioned, right or left arm dominance can mask other adaptations. In the example of a short right leg producing an elevated left shoulder (the "S" shape), the shoulder elevation deriving from the leg-length difference will tend to be increased in a left-handed person due to the greater development of the shoulder and neck muscles on the left side. In contrast, a right-handed person may show perfectly level shoulders, even with a shorter right leg. Here, one adaptation is balanced with another so that there is no easily discernible visible difference. Despite appearing symmetrical to the casual observer, such a person may still suffer from neck or back pain from the asymmetrical distribution of forces around the lower back and neck due to the leg-length inequality. Visual inspection cannot be guaranteed to reveal all that one needs to know to solve problems. An additional complicating factor is the question of whether an observed short leg is structural (left/right differences in key bones in the lower half of the body) or *induced*. The latter can occur as an adaptation to a *scoliosis* (lateral curvature of the spine), through tension held in particular muscles for a variety of reasons, or shortness in muscles due to previous injury. Doing the tests outlined in chapter one will stretch the involved muscles, and reexamining your shape will often reveal that the lateral curves are reduced.

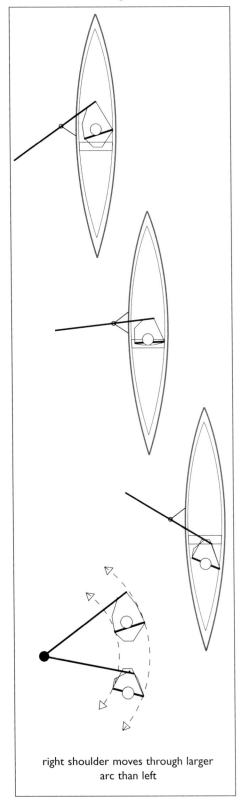

Schematic of rowing

right shoulder moves through larger arc than left

Adding another layer to the argument

To the notion of structural asymmetry needs to be added the idea (another layer in effect) of functional symmetry—a comparison of symmetry of function, derived from a consideration of both structural and functional aspects. A "function" used in this sense is a "global" property of a person, such as the ability to bend at the hip, or the capacity to rotate at the waist. The term global refers to those macro-scale properties of the whole person that arise through the properties of a number of smaller parts—bones, nerves, ligaments, muscles and so on. Any global property cannot be directly traced to any single subsystem but arises from the particular arrangement of these systems, together with their individual properties.

All these functions are overlaid with acquired patterns of movement, mental attitude and so on—all the possible factors that contribute to the way the body functions at any given time. Consider, for example, a "sweep" rower who rows in a team of four or eight people. In this sport, the body's power is transmitted to the oar through an arc of considerable size. See the illustration. The right arm and shoulder (on the outside of this arc) travels further than the left. All the muscles of the right-hand side of the spine contract through a wider arc and experience greater loads. A significant component of rotation is thus added to the fundamental extension movement of rowing. Over time, if the athlete always rows on the same side of the boat, the muscles of the back develop unevenly. This means that even a rower who is perfectly balanced (structurally speaking) will acquire (and display) uneven function, both in terms of flexibility and strength. This alone can contribute significantly to back pain. Even if you are not a competitive athlete, similar movements can affect you. For example, if you play golf or tennis, or always turn your head strongly each day only in one direction (which side do you look over as you back the car out of the garage each day?), you are likely to develop similar asymmetry.

Testing functional flexibility does not require a complex set of tests to be administered by an expert. It merely refers to a selection of the stretching exercises covered in chapter one. The key functions to be tested for are (with respect to back pain) right and left lateral flexion and right and left rotation of the spine. Because of the lack of symmetry between the front and back halves of the body, no absolute standards can be suggested for comparisons of flexion and extension in the individual case. However, each half of the body should be the same or very similar, so regardless of your flexibility in absolute terms, the flexibility of each half of the trunk (in both the movements mentioned), and each arm and leg should ideally be the same.

There is no necessary relation between trunk flexion and extension (forward and backward bending). A person who is unusually flexible in extension may be anywhere between flexible and stiff in flexion. Beyond stating that you should improve your flexibility within the limits of your strength, it is impossible to specify desirable limits for these functions. The spine is far more flexible bending backwards than forwards (apart from its structure, the ribs obstruct flexion of the thoracic spine, and the chest blocks forward movement of the chin, thus limiting flexion of the cervical spine). Maximally flexible individuals can exhibit up to 110 degrees of flexion and up to 140 degrees of extension (Kapandji, 1974, vol. III, p. 44). Note that these figures are estimated with respect to the plane of the bite, and include the possible movements of the entire spine. If anything, Kapandji underestimated the possible flexibility of the lumbar spine in extension (he gives 35 degrees). His illustration of a common yoga pose on the same page supports this objection. In any case, the trained individual has considerable freedom of movement available. Within limits, improving the range of movement of the individual parts of the spine (providing there is sufficient strength to support the movement) will make the body feel looser and more relaxed. It will also help the body to settle into a form that is closer to the minimum-energy configuration.

When we consider the spine from behind, we can be more certain in our analysis. In general, right and left lateral flexion should be the same, because the structures involved in these movements are symmetrical. Right and left rotation, while involving additional structures from the anterior–posterior plane that we admitted have no necessary symmetry, also involve the symmetrical plane in each rotational range. Because half of these additional structures are involved in rotation to each side, these movements should also be symmetrical, but in all the testing we have done, we have never found symmetry in these movements in anyone who suffers back pain. The degree of total movement in this plane may suggest additional checking of the degree of freedom of the hip flexors and extensors. For example, if you cannot lie face-up and press the lower back flat onto the floor with the legs held straight, it is likely that your hip flexors are too tight, and this will contribute to certain kinds of back pain.

Looking at the region of the upper back and neck, we expect to see a balanced structure. Things to look for include the way the head is carried on the neck, how the neck is carried on the shoulders, and the elevation of respective shoulders. Consider whether your thoracic spine is straight. As with the lumbar spine, a slight forward inclination of the upper body can reveal a lateral curve, particularly if the back is illuminated from the side. Look at how the arms are carried. Is one arm rotated more inwardly than the other? This may indicate that the front shoulder muscle or the biceps muscle on this side is tighter than on the other. If there is no problem with the arm or shoulder, this difference is merely something to keep an eye on. If there is a problem, these muscles should be looked at first.

The main exercises to test your functional flexibility are (in order of importance) right and left lateral flexion of the spine (treat the neck as part of the spine), and right and left rotation of the whole spine. The neck and the lower back may be tested separately. Follow this by testing hip flexion (the hamstring group) and hip extension (the hip flexors). If the latter appears markedly deficient, also test *quadriceps* flexibility, because we have found a high correlation with tight hip flexors—this may be found on one or both sides. If lateral flexion or rotation of the neck is found to be impaired, test shoulder flexibility, especially movements which stretch the front shoulder muscles and the long head of the biceps muscle. Do not test extension movements of the spine (including the neck) if there is any acute pain, because extension movements tend to aggravate this condition.

The keys to good posture are ease and efficiency. First and foremost, your posture needs to be pain-free and feel "easy," effortless and graceful. Secondly, the form of the body at any time needs to be efficient, or require a minimum of effort to support. Looking at this another way, good posture also allows the strength of the body to be used easily. It also facilitates the widest distribution of forces and hence enables the body in the most general sense. For this reason, there is not simply one kind of good posture. Different proportions and different personal histories make an absolute or universal determination of good posture impossible. Your task is to work on your own body to make it work as well as it can and to define your own best posture. Working with your body in the ways described will facilitate the unconscious acquisition of this most important attribute. Before turning to the experiences of the workshops we have been running around Australia nationally over the last eighteen months, I wish to consider the idea of cause (and the search for cause) itself.

Shortcomings with the idea of cause

We are used to the language of causality—that a particular effect is caused by something. Cause is familiar to us and shapes our way of thinking about the world. However, the usefulness of the ordinary idea of cause has limitations, and it is even possible that the very search for the cause of a particular illness may constrain solutions. Back pain is a good example of the problems of establishing the relation between symptom and cause. As mentioned previously, western medicine considers vertebral pathology to be the main cause of back pain. Here, "pathology" is used as shorthand for a range of deviations from normal, from abnormalities of the vertebrae to disease of the vertebral structures.

However, there are two problems in tracing cause in this common illness. The first problem is that back pain is widely described in the literature as having a *multifactorial aetiology* (many causal factors). The answer to the question of whether a potential cause should be considered cumulative, passive, or even countervailing, with respect to other coexisting causes, is far from clear. The first difficulty is to determine which cause of the multiple possible causes is likely to be the most important. Rules such as Occam's razor (that one is bound to choose the simplest explanation that fits the evidence) provide a useful constraint. The second problem is whether or not orthodox western medicine has a treatment for the particular cause identified. This problem suggests a practical relation between the ascription of "pathology" (as a label for a cluster of characteristics) and the prescription of treatment. The relation also partly explains medicine's tendency to define illness in terms of those attributes of the problem which are identifiable by the current technology (such as radiology, MRI or CAT scans, for example) and basing treatment on the results. As mentioned, these techniques do not "see" muscles.

Determining the cause of your problems is useful for both selecting and monitoring treatment, but which cause do you select? Considering our ongoing example, the short leg and its role in back pain, why do practitioners not focus attention on what might be its cause? And what of the cause that gave rise to it? In fact, every cause has a cause—how far back do you go in your analysis? This is one problem. Another is the problem of causes accompanying causes (the typical multifactorial or multicausal illness)—which do you select for treatment? What is the relationship between these multiple causes? Do their effects compound, does one counteract another, or is one possible cause nullified by another cause? Let us consider the short-leg syndrome as an example.

When one leg is shorter than the other, the normal curves of the spine in the sagittal plane may be subtly reproduced in the coronal plane, as we have discussed. This adaptation to uneven loads on the pelvis enables us to balance, through distribution of the asymmetric forces produced around the sacrum. Assuming the common "S"-shaped adaptation, a person with a slightly shorter right leg (with consequent tilting of the pelvis), will thus carry his or her left shoulder on the outside of a gently rightward curving thoracic spine (as seen from behind) if no other factors are present. This lateral curve (accompanied by additional development of the muscles on its convex side) may be a *cumulating* cause of neck pain in a left-handed person or a *countervailing* cause in a right-handed person. This is because of the increased muscular development (and usually increased tension) of the *trapezius* and *levator scapulae* muscles on the side of the dominant arm. In a right-handed person, the effects of these asymmetrical developments may well balance—with no net significance for middle back pain or neck pain. In a left-handed person, the effects may compound and cause middle back or neck pain through facet joint compression, segmental nerve impingement, muscle tension, or other mechanisms. External factors such as the uneven muscular development caused by an asymmetric sport (golf, for example) may be cumulative or countervailing causes for similar reasons. For these reasons, focusing on function is the best way to consider the problem, both diagnostically and curatively.

Workshop experiences

My group has been conducting public workshops around Australia for the last eighteen months: one-day intensives for individuals who suffer neck and back problems and three-day intensives for practitioners who deal with these problems. Approximately 1,200 people have attended the individuals' workshops. The majority were long-term neck or back pain sufferers, all of whom had sought treatment previously from other practitioners, including physiotherapists (around 30%), doctors (35%), chiropractors and osteopaths (over 60%), and a variety of other practitioners. Most had sought treatment from more than one kind of practitioner. In the vast majority, any relief had been temporary (a day to a few days the most common response) and most participants expressed the desire to learn how to look after themselves, preferably freeing themselves from the necessity of seeking regular treatment. The only stipulation made of the participants was that they were mobile enough to walk into the workshops. Many brought the results of various diagnostic technologies. The workshops begin by asking the participants to describe their problem, what treatments had been sought, and what results experienced.

The assumption of the workshops is that the main sources of dysfunction (reduction in range of movement) and pain are the muscles of the body. The further assumption is that the pain is a combination of inaccurate body image (by this I mean that the stretch reflex is triggered inappropriately early in the range of movement, for a variety of reasons including protection patterns held over from an earlier trauma or other causes) and muscle tension, also deriving from a variety of causes, which we have discussed above. Following the structural analysis described in chapter one, stretching exercises (or parts of standard exercises) were used diagnostically to compare key functions. In the vast majority, the location of the problem pain is in the tighter of paired muscles. Whether this tightness is a result of pathology or whether tightness should be considered a pathology is an open question. Treatment consisted of the recommended precise stretching exercises, using the Contract-Relax (C–R) approach to increase range of movement, to reduce muscular pain, and to remake dysfunctional patterns and body image.

The most important apparent causes of back pain identified have been an actual leg-length difference, with or without tight *iliopsoas*. These muscles have been found to be tight in absolute terms (45%, using the standard test, following Kendall, 1971) or tighter on one side (55%; this includes a proportion of the previous figure). In order of frequency, the muscles in which pain is experienced are *quadratus lumborum* (the most common) and *erector spinae* (less common) when the pain is lower back and one-sided, between the hip and the spine (around 60%), the fascia into which *latissimus dorsi* inserts when the pain is lower (10%; including apparent sacro-iliac joint and ligament pain), *gluteus medius* and *minimus* if the pain is high and deep in the buttock, and *piriformis,* about which more below. In middle back pain, the most common location is in one or both of the pairs of extensor muscles (a large number of muscles comprise this group) and the *rhomboids.* With respect to neck pain, the most significant source of pain is *levator scapulae,* and the most important cause of referred pain in the arm and hand has been found to be the *scalenus* group.

One further assumption is that pathology identified in any reports brought along by the participants is not of the severity wherein surgical intervention is either recommended or likely to be effective. Most participants with sciatica, for example, have been told that the severity of any identified pathology did not indicate surgery. A small number (4 individuals; n=1,180) were seeking to avoid surgery. A substantial number (110 individuals; n=1,180) had been informed that no significant pathology could be identified to explain their problems, and the most common recommendation in these cases was to seek the services of a pain control clinic, or to use relaxation techniques or similar to learn to live with the pain.

The workshops are providing evidence to support the claim that leg-length difference is significantly overrepresented among back and neck pain sufferers, compared to the results of various studies done over the last 20 years. As discussed, the standard figures are that 10–14% of the population have a leg-length difference of 9–10mm or more. From the raw data provided in the radiological studies considered above, calculation shows that differences in leg length of 5mm or more are found in over 50% of the *general* population.

The workshops have shown that uneven development of the lumbar and thoracic muscles is common. Few of the attendees have been athletes, and on questioning the vast majority of participants did not regularly engage in unusual asymmetrical activities, any more than the demands of daily life. The inference here is that the body can be considered a "map" of the forces that have acted upon it, and that a visual comparison of the shape of the muscles permits conclusions to be drawn about how the individual's body uses itself.

At the workshops we group the participants into pairs. We begin with a visual inspection of the whole body (with only the lumbar muscles and lower limbs exposed), looking for ankle pronation, symmetry of hips with respect to shoulders, level of shoulders, and placement of head. Comparison of left and right waist indentations are useful for women. We then ask the participant to stand with a small plastic block of about half an inch (6 millimeters) thickness under each heel in turn. When the block is under the longer leg, the distortion to the symmetry is obvious, both to observers and the participant. When placed under the shorter leg, the patient looks and feels more balanced.

Around 75% displayed a slight to dramatic tilting of the pelvis. If the use of the block causes equal or similar distortion to the shape of the body on both sides, no significant difference is the conclusion. The most remarkable aspect of the testing process is that after a few pairs of people have been tested, the other participants of the workshop are able to identify this asymmetry without prompting—this asymmetry is common, but we do not generally look for it, and it remains unidentified. A heel lift is recommended where necessary.

With respect to asymmetrical morphology of the muscles of the lumbar and thoracic spine, one additional point needs to be made. Over the 10 years of running stretching exercise classes at the Australian National University (around 200 new students per semester), we have found an inverse relationship between strength and flexibility. For example, in the normal healthy pain-free adult, the standard tests of shoulder flexibility have revealed that the vast majority of right-handed people have reduced shoulder joint flexibility in all planes of movement. As far as the whole body is concerned, if the flexibility of any paired muscle group is measured, we have found that (in the individual who does not include stretching exercises in their normal routine) the stronger or visibly better developed muscle usually tests tighter. With respect to individuals who display asymmetrical muscular development following pelvic obliquity, the pain has been found to be located in the tighter of a pair of muscles.

Following structural analysis, five tests of functional flexibility are performed by the group, in pairs. Working in pairs facilitates good form in the tests, and teaches the participants how to correct the body's natural tendency to avoid stretching the muscles that are tight. The tests are right/left rotation, right/left hip flexion (with both bent and straight legs), right left/lateral flexion, left/right hip extension, and left/right *piriformis*. If the attendee complains of sciatica, a straight leg-lifting test (the partner version of exercise 11) is performed first and followed with the *piriformis* test. The straight leg-lifting test is then performed a second time. About half the sciatica sufferers report immediate improvement, both in pain reduction and freedom of movement in the hip.

The most-often found pattern of flexibility associated with a leg-length difference are that buttock and hamstring muscles test looser on the shorter leg, rotation of the lumbar spine looser when the shorter leg is taken to the floor in the lying rotation test, lateral flexion is tighter *away* from the short leg side, and the hip flexors are tighter on the short leg side. These patterns are not immutable, however, and we advise attendees to identify their own patterns and treat these, by beginning their stretching workouts with the tighter of the pairs, and finishing with the tighter pair and thus doing more work for these muscles over time.

Although it is commonly believed that tight hamstring muscles can cause back pain, the mechanism through which this occurs is not clear. Kapandji notes that as the hamstrings contract, they flatten the lumbar curve (vol. III, p. 106), so their action militates against other muscles' actions that increase the curve—an increased curve often being cited as a possible cause of back pain. The reason hamstring muscles are correctly implicated in back pain is that if they are particularly tight, much forward bending in normal life is achieved by flexion of the spine (flattening of the lumbar curve) rather than at the hip joint. Bending this way accentuates the shearing forces already present at the L5–S1 interface (the *lumbosacral* joint), increasing wear and tear, and predisposing the patient to disc injury at this level. Bending this way also requires the extensors of the spine to contract or lengthen under load which can cause fatigue or muscle spasm, especially if combined with rotation. These effects may occur even when the hamstring muscles

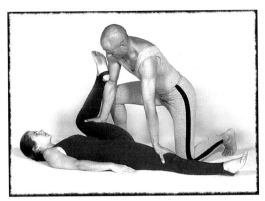

Test of hip flexion

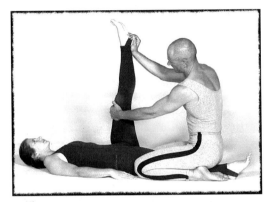

1 Test hamstring length then first C-R

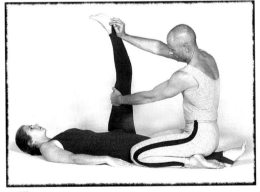

2 Second C-R

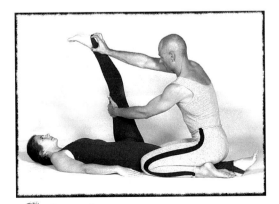

3 Restretch

are sufficiently loose to permit efficient movement, through poor movement patterns (that is, by bending forward from the lumbar spine rather than from the hips). Short hamstrings may even be the *result* of an exaggerated lumbar curve (Twomey and Taylor, 1994, p. 60).

Of perhaps more interest is a *comparison* of hamstring tightness. The hamstring muscles of the shorter leg usually test looser anteroposteriorly, as does the hip joint of the shorter leg in this plane. Test results (exercise 11) may thus add weight to the determination of a short leg. If you find that the exercise tests show a pattern confirming what might be expected with a shorter leg and yet your partner did not find a difference in the standing test, you may wish to do the leg-length test again. A difference in hamstring flexibility in a patient who is an athlete may be significant for other reasons. This is because of the unequal stresses produced around the sacrum during training and during competition. This seems particularly significant for distance runners.

In chapter one, I mentioned that I would return to the partner version of exercise 11 and explain why this must be done carefully. Practitioners use a similar movement to determine whether there is disc or nerve root involvement in your back pain, called the straight leg-lifting (or raising) test, or SLLT. The leg must be moved into the test position extremely carefully (that is, slowly and gently) because the nerve roots are pulled out from the intervertebral foramina for up to 12 millimeters at the L5 level during the test. Incautious elevation of the leg can produce sufficient traction on the nerve to rupture some of the involved axons (nerve fibers) if they are unable to be pulled through this space, which may result in paralysis (Kapandji, 1974, vol. III, p. 126).

Pain felt at the back of the leg between the buttock and the area just below the back of the knee in the hamstring test may be a false positive sign in this test, however. To distinguish between tight hamstrings and nerve involvement, find the point in the range of movement in the test where the pain is first felt. Then perform the two contractions described in exercise 11 while your partner maintains the leg's position. Wait for a breath in and as you breathe out, ask your partner to very gently elevate the leg. If the pain was caused by tight hamstrings, the leg will go past the initial point to a new stretch position, perhaps into the normal range. If nerve root involvement is present it will not. May I remind you that these tests must be done extremely carefully. Hoppenfeld suggests dorsiflexing the ankle (moving the ball of foot towards knee) at the point pain is first felt. If pain is not experienced in the back, the test pain is probably due to tight hamstrings (Hoppenfeld, 1976, p. 256). My experience suggests that adding this stretch is quite likely to increase the pain felt all the way along the back of the leg. This is often due to a tight *gastrocnemius* (calf) muscle. Additionally, any restriction to the small movements of the sciatic nerve through the calf muscles required by this test (sometimes referred to as "nerve tethering") may also give a false positive. If retesting after stretching *gastrocnemius* (see exercise 30) shows that the leg moves higher than before, suspect this possibility.

We have found tight hip flexors correlated with central low back pain, and a single tight hip flexor correlated with one-sided *quadratus lumborum* pain. As mentioned, the tighter hip flexor is usually found on the short leg side; this is the least reliable of the patterns, but found in over 60% of participants. Tight hip flexors have been found to be highly correlated with an increased lumbar lordosis, often in association with bilateral tightness of *quadratus lumborum* and *erector spinae.* If the hip flexors (*iliopsoas* and sometimes *rectus femoris*) are tight, the leg will not extend past the line of the body (as is needed when walking, for example) without rotation of and/or anterior tilting of the pelvis. A suggested mechanism for pain in these patients is increased pressure on the facet joints together with the muscular causes mentioned. Lumbar flexion exercises usually provide immediate relief of this kind of pain. Long-term tightness may contribute to increased *kyphosis* and additional compensating cervical lordosis, caused by the body's need to carry its weight over the balance point. Effective stretching of the hip flexors is difficult unless the trunk is braced, as stretching these muscles extends the lumbar spine and frequently elicits the participant's pain.

The functional relationship between the respective strengths and flexibilities of *iliopsoas* and *quadratus lumborum* is not adequately researched. In addition to their role in shaping the lumbar curve, these muscles play a critical role in the rotational stability of lumbar vertebrae. *Iliopsoas* has fibers that attach to the anterior processes of each lumbar vertebra. *Quadratus lumborum*'s fibers attach to the posterior processes of the lumbar vertebrae, as well as having fine fibers spanning the distance between the iliac crest and the last rib. Ideally, the forces generated by these muscles should balance, both at the level of the individual vertebra as well as the lumbar curve as a whole. Alternatively, if these forces occur sequentially (as with any movement), the forces should balance over time. Balance thus needs to be considered in dynamic terms in addition to what static tests may reveal. The forces produced by the energetic movements of sport or energetic exercise are far greater than those typically produced in static situations. For a fuller causal picture, the particular demands you place on your body need to be considered.

From the research done by the manipulative therapies, we can assume that ideal position of a vertebra can be disturbed reasonably easily. Weakness or tightness in a single set of the connecting muscle fibers may be sufficient to slightly rotate one vertebra with respect to its neighbors. On the larger scale, our work suggests that excessive lumbar lordosis can be caused by shortness of the *iliopsoas* group (through the pull on the anterior surfaces of the transverse processes), and that the resulting anterior tilt of the pelvis is accompanied by shortness of both *quadratus lumborum* and the extensors of the spine. Back pain is often blamed on weakness in the abdominal muscles (whose contractions tend to flatten the lumbar curve). However, tight *iliopsoas* can easily overwhelm even strong abdominal muscles for strength and leverage reasons, and *iliopsoas* can cause additional extension to the spine during walking and other normal movements. This is

As leg extends, hip joint ligaments tighten around neck of femur

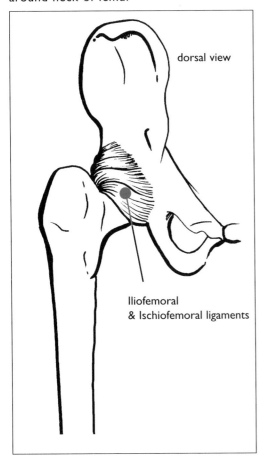

dorsal view

Iliofemoral & Ischiofemoral ligaments

partly due to the length of the legs, which are levers of great length that can easily exert enough force through inflexible *iliopsoas* to affect the lumbar curve. Tests show that only very rarely are the abdominal muscles strong enough to stretch *iliopsoas*. Remember that the conventional "sit-up" exercise (where the whole back is lifted off the floor, as opposed to the "crunches" and curls we recommend) strengthens *iliopsoas* more than the abdominal groups. The common prescription of these exercises to strengthen the abdominals usually worsens the initial imbalance—that is, *iliopsoas* becomes even stronger than the abdominals through this activity.

During walking and running, all the leg muscles are used to move the body over the foot. As the leg passes the midline of the body, inflexible *iliopsoas* pulls the lumbar curve into further extension or rotates the pelvis in the transverse plane, following the leg if there is insufficient flexibility. In the muscularly balanced and sufficiently flexible person, even the much more exaggerated action of running does not appreciably change the lumbar curve, as slow-motion photography has shown. Although these effects are likely to be exacerbated by a leg-length difference, they can be present even when the legs are of identical lengths. A muscular imbalance can arise through use patterns, injury, or the like. For this reason any functional imbalance must be treated if found—even in the absence of structural differences.

There is one factor that complicates this analysis. Most anatomists agree that the lumbar curves are an adaptation facilitating the transition from four legs to two in our distant past. In the "on all fours" position (on the hands and knees) the anterior ligaments of the hip (*iliofemoral*, *pubofemoral* and *ischiofemoral*) are relaxed, and run roughly coincident with the neck of the femur, similar to quadrupedal mammals. In humans standing in the normal erect posture, these ligaments are under moderate tension. This skeletal position would correspond to strong extension of the hip joint in quadrupedal mammals. Any movement of the leg back from the midline from the erect position strongly tightens these ligaments, which are by this stage wound around the neck of the femur. These ligaments are considerably less extensible than *iliopsoas*. We have found, however, that *iliopsoas* is the limiting factor in the great majority of people demonstrating reduced range of movement in this area.

Another often unsuspected cause of back and hip pain is one of the external hip rotators, *piriformis*. In about one-fifth of the population, the peroneal branch of the sciatic nerve passes directly through this muscle rather than passing below it (Travell & Simons, 1992, vol. II, p. 186 ff.). Recent research suggests that smaller branches of parts of the sciatic nerve can pierce *piriformis* as well, one source claiming that this is found in up to 37% of the general population (Chiba *et al.*, 1994). If this muscle is in spasm or simply very tight, enough clamping force can be produced on parts of the sciatic nerve to cause pain in the muscles behind the hip joint and sciatic pain down the back of the leg. Typical histories include long periods of sitting. This pain can feel the same as sciatica caused by disc impingement. If the patient has disc pathology, a diagnosis of nerve-impingement induced sciatica may be made without there being any causal relationship between the pathology and the symptoms.

Choice of bed

The recommendation is commonly made that a firm bed is the best kind for people with neck or back problems. This recommendation needs to be considered in relation to both your shape and your body weight. A firm base is desirable in any case, but one patient noted that a sagging base provided some relief for his back pain, largely caused by an excessive lumbar lordosis. I believe that one needs to choose a mattress or other support that deforms sufficiently to permit the buttocks to rest far enough below the surface of the rest of the bed that the lumbar spine feels comfortable. Accordingly, if you are a light person, you will find a too-firm mattress uncomfortable. If you have well-developed (prominent) buttocks, you too may need a softer mattress than is usually recommended. However, these remarks will need to be modified if you are relatively heavy. Overall, I think that the body needs to be supported in such a way as to allow the spine to be held in its most comfortable position. You will need to consider also the shape of the spine while lying on your side: ideally, in this position the spine should be as close to straight as possible. This means that a woman with wider hips might need a softer mattress than a man of similar weight, but with broader shoulders and narrower hips. A compromise in firmness that permits the best possible face-up and lying-side positions is desirable.

As far as neck pain is concerned, my experience is that you need a pillow that is sufficiently firm and thick when compressed by the weight of the head to hold the head as close to the neutral position as possible in the side-lying position. I suggest that no pillow be used when lying face-up. If you go to sleep in the lying face-up position, you may care to try to go to sleep with the pillow behind you, within grasping distance. Patients have told me that if they go to sleep this way, they reach for the pillow automatically during the night when they roll over on their side.

Chapter five considers relaxation and its role in the healing process, and describes a simple method to help you reduce the effects of stress.

RELAXATION TECHNIQUES

Practical Stress Management seminars

Most of this chapter is drawn from the Practical Stress Management seminars I do for private companies and senior and middle management levels of government. Usually slotted into the middle of a week of workshops devoted to more conventional management techniques, these seminars have been received extremely well. In them, I use a number of the most important exercises presented in this book to show each manager precisely (and dramatically) where he or she actually holds tension resulting from daily stress. The whole seminar lasts three hours, but in this chapter I present a slightly more formal version of the last thirty minutes, which teaches a quick way of learning how to relax. Do not be put off by the term "quick." The method combines elements of old and new techniques, and is more effective than any single approach I have come across to date. It is now accepted that one's mental state can be altered by changing one's physical state, and the converse is also true (see Achterberg, 1985, in the *Further Reading* list). To this point in the book, we have dealt with the physical almost exclusively, but it is now time to consider the mental–physical nexus.

In passing, it may be useful to contrast the attitudes of the participants of these courses with those of our students in the *Posture & Flexibility* classes. Whether a defense against appearing vulnerable in front of their peers or whether a function of a typical mix of personality traits displayed by managers, the suggestion that learning how to relax will be directly useful is usually met with skepticism, especially by the male participants. Evidently, most managers believe (or affect the belief when they are in these groups) that non-mainstream medicine or practices are somehow strange, and unlikely to be useful to the modern manager. I am usually greeted by a sea of raised eyebrows, folded arms and similar body language when I first enter the seminar room—a tough audience, in other words.

When I began giving these seminars, I used to mount what I considered to be unassailable arguments, supported by evidence drawn from different areas of research, and all converging on the position I was advocating. With an academic audience, this strategy may have succeeded, but it failed completely with the more pragmatic managers. Accordingly, I gave thought to how one might quickly and thoroughly convince an audience of the worth of the ideas and techniques presented.

I decided to use a neck exercise as a demonstration in the first minutes of the presentation. I use the neck side bend (exercise 17), complete with the contraction and relaxation parts. All participants' necks move closer to the shoulder after doing this, and I then ask them to repeat for the other side, comparing left with right. By this time (two minutes later) audience attention and participation is always 100%. The old adage that you can take a horse to water but you cannot make it drink is true, as far as it goes. A different approach is to make that horse feel thirsty. I use this approach with relaxation techniques I teach as the concluding part of these seminars as well. I offer no explanation, and go directly to the script (at the end of this chapter), so the participants can *feel* the value of the techniques. Here though, before we get to the script I shall present a brief discussion of the whys and wherefores of relaxation.

Why relax?

Stress is a much-used and abused term in the languages of medicine and that activity known as "human resource management." Originally an engineering term, *stress* was popularized in medicine by the pioneer of this research, Dr. Hans Selye. Selye conceived of stress as those aspects of the environment that provoke a response in the organism. He divided stress into *eustress*, or good stress, and *distress*, which includes the familiar meaning. The originality of Selye's research lies mainly in his uncovering of the physical processes that mediate these stresses—the adrenal glands and their associated hormones—and his demonstration that the two types of stress (perceived so differently by the individual) have remarkably similar physiological effects on the body (Selye, 1978).

The effects of stress have been labelled as the "fight or flight" response. They are characterized by physical and psychological changes such as increased respiration and pulse rates, increased blood pressure, increased sympathetic nervous system activity, and increased feelings of "pressure." Physiologists assume that these responses prepare the organism (for these responses are not limited to humans) for fighting or evading danger in the environment. Further, they assume that modern humans are the result of past evolutionary forces, and hence very likely to be the progeny of organisms who were successful in coping with these kinds of pressures. However, these responses may well be inappropriate in the modern office environment. This change to our normal environment is the crux of Selye's research. If one does not fight or flee, the crucial question is what happens to the body if this response (with all its accompanying hormones, increased blood sugar and other metabolic changes) is repeatedly activated and not used?

Without doubt, one common result is the disease known as the "silent killer"—*hypertension*, or permanently elevated blood pressure. This condition is considered to be a major predisposing cause of many fatal heart conditions and similar serious diseases. Everyone is aware of the momentary muscular effects of being frightened or angry (immediately increased tension in all the muscles of the body). However, the main effect of the repeated activation of this response is permanently elevated tension in the muscles of the body. Elevated muscle tension may even be the primary cause of hypertension. Either way, those muscles that are "prestressed" for one reason or another are precisely those muscles of concern to us here—the neck and back muscles. I believe that our evolutionary inheritance, coupled with a sedentary lifestyle, is one of the main reasons neck and back pain is so commonplace.

Fortunately, there is a complementary physiological and psychological response, tentatively named the "relaxation response" (Benson, 1976), which can be cultivated simply by everyone. This response appears to be controlled by the *hypothalamus*, just as is the fight or flight response. The effects of the relaxation response are the opposite of those of the fight or flight response, and also include the effect of reduced tension in the muscles of the body. It is not at all clear why most people are more effective at mobilizing the fight or flight response rather than the relaxation response, but I suspect that evolutionary pressures favored the former and not the latter. The relaxation response—which everyone demonstrates to some degree—can be vastly enhanced and actively used to counter the stress of life.

For the sufferer of neck or back pain, learning how to access this response may be used in the short term to cope with the pain or discomfort of an attack (by helping the relevant muscles relax). It can also be used in the medium to long term to increase the "headroom" between the normal state of the muscles and the kind of tension which predisposes you to an attack of neck or back pain. Together with the stretching and strengthening exercises, improving the relaxation response forms a highly efficient multi-stranded approach to alleviating the problem.

Relaxation method

I shall use Benson's four elements leading to "the elicitation of the Relaxation Response" (p.78 ff.) to structure my recommendations for your practice. In passing, it should be noted that Benson's book outlines the major research done in various techniques said to lead to a relaxed or meditative state. He found that all the disciplines considered—regardless of cultural origin—shared many common methods and resulted in virtually identical physiological states. For an excellent and not-too-technical review, I recommend this book for further reading on this fascinating subject.

The first requirement is a quiet environment in which to do one's practice. Although a quiet place is useful to learn how to feel this relaxation response (and then how to create it at will), it is not essential once you have learned. It is commonplace in Japan for people to meditate on trains, which are very noisy places indeed. An interesting aspect of this relaxed state (and one of the ways you will know you have achieved it) is that, although sounds around you seem further away, you can still attend to their essential content, but in a rather more detached way than usual. In normal daily life, you should find a time and a place where you are not likely to be disturbed. Before dinner or before sleep are especially good times for many people. And for the reasons given earlier, it is best to seclude yourself from your spouse and children. A three-year-old child regards the prone body as a direct invitation to crawl and play, and this will not help your practice! Similarly, pull the telephone connection out of the wall. You will need only ten to fifteen minutes of peace and quiet.

Benson's second element is "a mental device," like repeating a sound to yourself, concentrating your gaze on a symbol, or concentrating on a feeling. The last recommendation I have found to be the most effective, and I shall expand on this point below. The third element is "a passive attitude," an "emptying of all thoughts and distractions from one's mind" (p.78). I spent a long time in Zen temples in Japan trying to do just this little thing. As any of you who have tried to do this will know, it is extremely hard to do. Being able to "empty the mind" is the mark of an expert, and is not the best advice for beginners who need another approach—in effect, something appropriate to *fill* the mind.

Benson's last element is "a comfortable position." Various sitting positions are the recommendations of both Zen and Yoga, although some sects' practitioners meditate while walking. Lying down is usually not recommended, in the belief that it often leads to sleep in the untrained individual. We are trying to find that mental and physical state where we seem to be hovering between wakefulness and sleep, and falling asleep is not desirable. In my experience, it is perfectly possible to meditate in any comfortable position. The recommendation about sitting in the lotus pose, for example, are completely inappropriate for all but experienced yoga practitioners. Until you can sit in this pose in perfect comfort for ten or fifteen minutes, the sensations in your legs are guaranteed to distract you from the purpose, deep relaxation. However, if you can sit in this pose for the required time, it is ideal because it locks the pelvis into a stable position and enables you to keep a straight back without effort.

My recommendations for practice are to lie stretched out face-up on the floor without a pillow, providing this is comfortable. The floor is better than a bed, because you do not want to drift off to sleep, and if you are lying on your bed the associations will be difficult for the mind and the body to ignore. If your back is sore, or if lying on the floor with the legs stretched out is uncomfortable, put a pillow or similar object under the knees to flex the legs. This will not detract from the effect we are seeking. Wear warm clothing or cover yourself with a blanket. Loosen any tight clothing, particularly collars and belts. Make sure that you do not need to go to the toilet in the next 15 minutes.

Place one hand flat on your chest and the other flat on your abdomen, above the navel. Many people do not breathe abdominally but breathe mostly into the top of the chest. Most physiologists believe that chest breathing is not optimally efficient, because it requires the "muscles of inspiration" (the *scalene* group, among others) to be used in addition to the diaphragm. These neck, shoulder and rib muscles are used together with the diaphragm when we are breathing really deeply, as might happen when you sprint for the bus or as you sit gasping in the bus recovering from the unaccustomed run, or when you are frightened. However, these muscles are not the ones to use when learning how to relax, partly because of the emotional states the body has learned to associate with their use. For this reason, when you begin practice, place your hands as suggested. As you breathe in, you will feel the hand over the navel rise as the abdomen is pressed out by the diaphragm contracting. Ideally, the hand on the chest should not move. If it does, try to feel how to breathe so that it does not (pressing the stomach *out* as you breathe in is a good way to start). Once you feel the difference, practice will be easy. Imagine the breath flowing deep into the abdomen while you try to feel it. Like many things, it is more a matter of awareness than the need to develop a special skill.

I do not share the common recommendation of having an object to dwell on or a sound (*mantra*) to chant. Of course, if you already practice this way successfully, please continue to do so. Obviously, a beginner will find it helpful to concentrate on something, and in place of an object or sound, I suggest you divide your concentration between two aspects of your practice, changing from one to the other as distracting thoughts occur. In this way, you will be able to combine two of Benson's elements in a new way to produce the desired effect.

To begin, lie as suggested and close your eyes. You may like to have soothing music on in the background, especially something repetitive and structured without dramatic passages. If you have recorded the script I suggest below, you can play it, either on headphones or on a stereo. Alternatively, you could record it with suitable music playing in the background. Concentrate on one part of the body, starting with the feet, in turn. Determine whether that part feels comfortable. If it does not, or if you are not sure whether it is as relaxed as it could be, make a small movement to bring the toes closer to each other and relax, letting the feet fall outwards. (In this case, the position of the feet is controlled by the hip muscles, but because the action of the hip joint produces movement of the feet, it is convenient to think of it as a foot movement.)

Next consider for a moment the sensation of how the foot position feels. The concentration is then shifted to the breath. Breathe in and out three times, not making any effort to control the breathing (that is, make no effort to slow or deepen the breathing). Here, we adopt a passive attitude of "seeing" the breath come into, and leave, the body. Concentrate on the many sensations accompanying this most familiar of activities, but of which we usually are completely unaware—the feeling of air flowing through the nose and down the throat, and so on. Feel the rise and fall of the abdomen. Following the three breaths, return your concentration to the body, to the next part in the sequence presented in the script. From this we return to the breath, each time using a slightly different way of breathing, which I explain in the script. Where the directions say to hold your breath in, keep the throat *open* as you do so, using the diaphragm to keep the air in your lungs. The way we normally hold the breath (throat closed and the breath's pressure felt against the throat) lifts the blood pressure, which we do not want. Where the directions say to hold the breath out, again keep the throat open, using the abdominal muscles to hold the breath out.

In this way, we are dividing the concentration between two distinct sets of feelings, each rich with sensation. Such concentration fills the brain with information—and hence stops the thoughts that normally rush into one's mind in the absence of thought. This is my way of emptying the mind. It is an active way of avoiding the normal distractions, and leads you into a relaxed state effortlessly and without frustration. The concentration span required in each breath phase is deliberately brief. Teaching this technique has shown that a beginner cannot maintain concentration easily on even a five-breath cycle (about twenty seconds). By swapping one's concentration relatively quickly between the two foci of attention, the mind does not have enough time to become bored or restless with any one set of thoughts. The experiences thus remain alive and consuming, with no space for distraction.

Guided visualization and healing the body

A new field of research in western medicine (not much more than ten years old) is called *psychoneuroimmunology* (psycho-neuro-immunology). It attempts to uncover the processes and relationships between psychological and physiological states. This research has revealed many mechanisms underlying our common-sense knowledge of how the world works, including the vitally important links between mood (mental state) and function (physiological process). The research strongly supports the claim—long made by many alternative health practitioners—that healing processes can be aided by thinking or feeling them into a more powerful response. I have included an excellent overview of this research in the *Further reading* list, a book called *Imagery in Healing*. Visualization of certain healing processes, when one is in an appropriately relaxed state, can speed the process. Similar visualization can be used to reduce the sensation of chronic pain or for other purposes. Accordingly, I have included a brief mention of useful visualizations for neck or back pain. A little imagination will allow you to adapt this script for other kinds of pain or to enhance performance of particular skills. Research has shown that this visualization fires the neurons involved (but at a sub-maximal level, so little movement of the involved muscles occurs), effectively rehearsing the skill without actually doing it. You may wish to expand this pain control section before you have the script recorded, adding specific details relevant to your situation.

Before we begin, let me remind you of the important check points:

Go to the toilet,

Take the telephone off the hook (or pull the connection from the wall),

Loosen any tight clothing and put on warm clothing.

A script for relaxation and visualization

(A note to the person recording the script: allow three to five seconds' pause between paragraphs as marked. Speak in a normal, but unhurried voice, without dramatic changes in intonation or pitch. Try to stay relaxed yourself as you record the script, and resist the common temptation to hurry your delivery.)

Lie down on a firm surface and close your eyes. We are going on a journey around the body, a journey designed to take you into a state of deep relaxation.

We'll begin with the feet. Adjust their position, using the smallest movements that have the desired effect. Bring the toes together a fraction, and let the feet fall to the sides. Wriggle the toes of the left foot a little until the foot feels completely comfortable. Now the right foot. Arch the foot and let it relax. Move the toes a little. Now try to feel both feet at the same time. Feel the weight of the feet press down onto the floor through the heels. Make sure that the heels feel comfortable.

Now, turn your attention to the breath. Begin by taking three relaxed breaths in and out. Don't try to slow or deepen your breathing. See and feel how the breath moves in and out of the body of its own accord. It is rhythmic and tidal. Feel the air move through the nose. See it going down the throat into the lungs. Feel it lifting your stomach under your hand. Feel how the breath flows, in and out.

Back to the body. Start with the right leg this time. Feel how the leg is resting on the floor, through the calf muscle. Often, this muscle is not as relaxed as it can be. To make sure, gently bring the toes of the right foot a small distance towards the right knee. Then let the foot relax to its most comfortable position. Now the left foot. Move the toes a little in the direction of the left knee, and let the left foot go. Feel the weight of both legs at the same time. You can feel their weight pressing onto the floor. Both legs feel relaxed, the heels and calf muscles resting comfortably on the floor.

For this next series of breaths, hold the breath *in* for a count of two. Keep the throat open, and hold the breath in for a count of two. Breathe in, and hold—count one, two. Now let the breath go out without forcing it in any way. See and feel the breath leaving the body. Repeat this cycle two more times. Breathe in. Hold—one, two. Let the breath go. Breathe in. Hold—one two. Let the breath go.

Turn your attention back to the body. From the legs, the next part of the body to contact the floor is the bottom. Make sure that the bottom is resting on the floor as comfortably as it can. Briefly and gently tighten the bottom muscles. Then let the muscles go completely soft. Now feel the weight of the bottom on the floor. Feel the weight of the whole of the legs, from the heels through the calf muscles to the bottom. This part of the body feels heavy now. As you become more relaxed it is normal for your body to feel heavier and heavier. It is a pleasant feeling. You are starting to feel somewhat detached from your surroundings, aware but a little distant.

This time, hold the breath *out* for a count of two. Breathe in normally. Don't hold the breath in this time. As soon as the lungs are full, breathe out. At the end of the breath out, breathe out a little more forcefully than before. Feel the stomach muscles tighten as you breathe out. Hold the breath out by using the abdominal muscles. Keep the throat open. Hold the breath out, and count—one, two. Relax, and let the air rush in. Feel its movement fill the lungs. Repeat this cycle two more times in your own time.

[If you are recording this script, pause for enough time for the next two breath cycles to be completed.]

Turn your attention back to the body. The next parts of the body to contact the floor are the back and the shoulders. Begin with the left shoulder. Very gently take its weight off the floor. Let it rest on the floor again. Now the right shoulder. Does it feel completely relaxed? If not, move it a small amount until it does. Does the part of your back on the floor feel completely comfortable? If not, move a small amount from side to side until it does. Now feel the weight of the whole body on the floor. You become aware of the weight of your body as you become more relaxed. It is a wonderful feeling of stillness, of being relaxed, of being comfortable.

This time, hold the breath both in and out. Breathe in. Hold the breath in for a count of one, two. Let the breath go out now. Feel the air going out of the body. At the end, breathe out the last part. Hold the breath out—one, two. In your own time, repeat this two more times. Do not force the breathing in or out. Do not try too hard. Relax with each breath out.

And now to the last part of the body, the head. Move the head a little from side to side to relax the neck muscles. Do they feel completely comfortable? You may need to tilt the head back a little, or it may need to come forward to feel completely comfortable on the floor. Now feel the enormous weight of the whole body, pressing on the floor from heels, calf muscles, through the bottom, the back and shoulders, and the head. Feel the body as one thing, pressing onto the floor. The body feels relaxed now, and it feels good. See yourself lying on the floor from above. You look completely relaxed.

Back to the breathing. This time, make no effort of any kind at all. Visualize the breath coming into the body. See it as a color. Which color doesn't matter. See the breath coming in through the nose, going down the throat, and into the lungs. Feel it going into the lungs. Feel the tummy rise. As you breathe out, imagine the breath as a different color. Choose one you like. Feel any tension remaining in the body going out with the breath. That's why it's now a different color. The more vividly you can visualize this, the more effective it will be. For the next cycle, concentrate your whole attention on five breaths in and out. If you find your attention wandering, turn it back to the body.

[If you are recording this script, pause long enough for four or five more breath cycles.]

And now back to the body. Feel the weight of the head on the floor again. Check to see whether the jaw muscles are holding tension. If you're not sure, lightly clench the teeth and let these muscles relax fully. Feel the muscles in the cheeks. Are they holding any tension? If so, lightly purse the lips, and let the face relax. Now the forehead. Frown briefly. Raise the eyebrows. Then let all the muscles of the face rest in their most relaxed positions. The face is a relaxed mask, now. It is serene. Feel the weight of the whole body. It is pressing on the floor. It feels very heavy. You feel completely relaxed and comfortable. Feel these sensations. This is what being relaxed feels like. It feels wonderful. You may feel as though you are floating. Or you may feel as though you are somehow removed from your surroundings. Sounds around you seem further away, and although you can still hear everything, the sounds do not disturb you.

Feel your breathing now. Imagine small waves breaking on a quiet beach. A little wave comes in, it lifts itself up, and breaks on the shore. As the water recedes, it makes a long hissing sound. It is a relaxing sound. It is a timeless sound. The movement of the waves is ceaseless. Your breath comes in as a little wave picks itself up. It goes out as the water recedes. Each breath out sounds like the water going out. Hear the sounds of the beach around you. Hear the faint cries of the seagulls, the sounds of the water. Feel a soft breeze on your face. You feel at peace with the world. Your body feels relaxed and heavy. You feel safe and secure. Concentrate on a few breaths, in and out.

This is the state of deep relaxation. You feel completely comfortable. Your body is healing itself as you relax in this state. The tension in your muscles is leaving the body with every breath out. It is now time to direct the healing processes to where they are needed. See your sore spots in your mind. Direct a flow of healing energy to these places. Imagine a colored light bathing these places. Imagine your body's healing processes at work. The more vividly you can see these things happening inside your body, the more effective they will be.

[If you are recording this script, pause for about thirty seconds. If you wish to adapt the script for sporting or skill performance, this is the place to insert the relevant cues. For example, if you wish to mentally rehearse a skill such as shooting baskets or putting, have the person recording the script say (for example) "Now see yourself shooting 20 baskets, perfectly." Mention in particular the aspects you wish to improve in as much detail as you can—the more detail, the better. Use positive language and ideas rather than negative ones.]

Your neck and back feel better than before, and you are going to feel better still as time goes on. Knots in your muscles are being smoothed away as tension leaves your body. The muscles of your neck and back feel more relaxed than they've ever been. These muscles feel warm, now. They feel comfortable, relaxed, and good. You know that tension prevents the body from healing itself. You are going to try to release tension from the body with each breath out, in your normal daily life.

Tell yourself it's good to be relaxed. It *feels* good to be relaxed. The stresses and strains of life do not affect me as much, now. And each time I practice, I improve. The state of deep relaxation comes to me faster than the last time I practiced, and the state of relaxation is deeper the more I practice. Each breath out relaxes you that tiny bit more. You are on a path which leads you to feeling more and more relaxed. Feel the feeling of deep relaxation.

[If you are recording this script, leave a long pause here—a minute or two.]

Now you want to rouse yourself from your deeply relaxed state. Some of the effects of deep relaxation will stay with you when you are fully awake. To come back to the normal world, breathe in deeply. Fill the whole of the chest. At the same time, raise your arms straight up and stretch them out behind you, back onto the floor. Press your toes away from you. Stretch your entire body. Breathe out as you bring your arms back to your sides. Stretch them out again, and breathe in fully. Bring the arms back to your sides, and relax. Sit up when you are ready.

Note: this script is available in a recorded form on audio cassette, called *The Relaxation Script.*

ACKNOWLEDGMENTS

The decision to write a book may be made lightly, but if my experience is anything to go by, finishing a book is an entirely different proposition altogether. And so it was with *Overcome Neck & Back Pain*— I am glad that I could not know how much sheer work it would take, because had I known I doubt that I would have taken the first steps. I am deeply grateful to the many people who have helped and encouraged me along the way.

My first debt of gratitude goes to my business partner, Paul Bottari. It is conventional to say things like "without his help, this book could not have been written." In this case, saying so is literally true. Paul provided me with financial support and friendship at many stages up to the final draft, and through to production and distribution of the first edition, published under the *BodyPress* colophon. As a brand-new publishing company, no one would give us financial credit, and we had to stretch ourselves to the limit before we saw a single copy of the book. Lindsay McKinnon of McPhersons Printing was very helpful in these early days.

In these acknowledgements, I wish to thank again the teachers of *Posture & Flexibility*, all of whom have contributed to the method as presented. I make a special thanks to Jennifer Cristaudo, my senior instructor, who teaches high school, edits books, and is mother to Anreus. Jennifer also modeled for many of the photographs and commented on an original draft. My brother and best friend, the scientist and author Dr. Greg Laughlin, deserves separate mention for reading an early draft and making suggestions that resulted in clearer argument. Olivia Allnutt, a public servant and an ex-gymnast, proofread all three editions. Thank you, indeed. Dr. Joe Hope and Dr. Kevin Moore, two of the most recent editions to the *P&F* team, both managed to finish their theses having started theirs after mine. Alan Richardson retired recently and he teaches the Over 40s *P&F* students. Working with these groups has refined the approach significantly and showed me time and again that age is no barrier to improvement. Pierre Le Count once claimed the distinction of being *Posture & Flexibility*'s least supple student (this is no longer the case). Matt Baker is a personal trainer and ex-member of the famous *Raiders* football team, and a man who demonstrates that weight-training and flexibility are not mutually exclusive. Matt was my training partner for a long time, too. Many other teachers who have come through our system are now found in various places away from our main teaching center at the Australian National University: David Moten (traveling, somewhere), Carol Wenzel is doing postdoctoral research at Davis University, Mark Donohue is a postdoctoral fellow in linguistics at Sydney University, Petra Boevink is a postdoctoral fellow at a research center in Scotland, Keiko Harada is now working in Japan's National Library, and Julie Netto is a doctoral candidate at Sydney University. Unfailingly cheerful and dedicated teachers, all. I commend these teachers to you, should you be fortunate enough to live in areas where classes are offered by them. And if you do not, make them an offer they can't refuse!

Kathy Sharpe (a good name for a photographer) came from Sydney to Canberra a number of times to take the photographs for the first edition, and Julia Topliss took the additional photos required for the present edition. When I received the original manuscript back from editor Dr. Michael Nunn, I could hardly see the words for the overlay of purple ink. However, after sober consideration of his liberal wielding of the purple pen (including some painful excisions), there was no doubt that the argument flowed better and the usages were more consistent. Any faults in the text remain mine alone, of course, although typos are the cats' responsibility. Jeremy Mears designed and manipulated all the images, text and photographs. *Overcome Neck & Back Pain* is still one of the few mainstream books that has been digitally constructed in its entirety, including all illustrations, photographs, text, and the cover, and which made all the changes to the three editions considerably less burdensome than they would have been otherwise. His website address is on the back title page.

Thank you Jon Attenborough, editor Lynne Segal, and David Roderick of *Simon & Schuster Australia* for your help in facilitating the second edition, and I look forward to a long association. For the present edition, my sincere thanks go to Jack Romanos of Viacom International who got the original book to an editors' meeting at Simon & Schuster, New York, and to *S&S* editor Caroline Sutton. I look forward to a long association with you, too.

I reserve a special mention for the most recent addition to the team of P&F teachers, and the woman who more than anyone else was responsible for getting the *Overcome Neck & Back Pain* workshops off the ground, Mrs. Sharon Clark. When the book received its initial television exposure here, Sharon called me to ask me to treat three members of her family. I declined, pleading pressure of my existing patient base and other work. I cannot recall just how many more times she called me with the same request with the same result, until one day in desperation she asked me what it would take to get me to her home town, Newcastle. I thought about this, and said that if she could find 20 people and a venue, I would come to her. An intense year's work later, which included 1,500 individuals and 350 practitioners (doctors, chiropractors, physiotherapists and massage therapists, with a sprinkling of Yoga, Pilates and Alexander technique teachers), I realize that this kind of persistence can move mountains. Thank you truly, Sharon.

Once they began, other people helped organize workshops for me, too. In Melbourne, Vickie Hatzis organized local workshops, and went on to organize practitioner workshops nationally. Steve Burton (a practitioner and yoga teacher) and Jackie Burton organized workshops in the Blue Mountains, and Michael Barron (helped ably by Ben and Steve) got the workshops together in Cairns. Many practitioners of different bodywork schools came to work with the *Posture & Flexibility* team throughout the year as a result of this exposure, and all helped to adapt and improve *P&F* as a system.

A great many readers of the two previous editions e-mailed me with feedback, and (as I'm fond of saying) if one is *truly* interested is assessing the worthwhilenss of an idea, failures are at least as significant as successes. Fortunately, the vast majoroty of e-mails detailed successes. Many of the improvements to this edition are the result of readers' suggestions. Thank you all.

On a personal note, I wish to acknowledge my intellectual debt to Dr. Richard Sylvan, who died last year. He was an inspiration to me, and chapter four grew partly out of my fascination with his *Relevant logic* system and his utter fearlessness in crossing traditional disciplinary boundaries. He hand-built houses in addition to systems of logic, and his insistence that individual systems need tying to the real world is an injunction that drives me still.

I wish to thank Megan and Ted for their respective special contributions to the original *BodyPress* edition.

Finally I want to thank you, reader, wherever you are: you are the final link in this long chain. But, please, do not be like a man who rushed up to me at the airport one day, exclaiming "I love your book!" I thanked him, and asked "Which exercises have you found the most useful?" He replied, "I haven't read it yet, but it's a beautiful book!" In one narrow sense, of course, we don't mind if you only use the book to prop open a door: a sale is a sale, after all. And some people who buy the book may keep it on the shelf somewhere until necessity leads them to it. But for the best results, don't just read the book, please *do the work!* Good luck.

References

Bolton, S. P., 1987. Similarities and differences between chiropractic and Osteopathy. J. Aust. Chiropr. Assoc., 17: 90–93.

Bradbeer, M., 1985. Nursing back from stress. Forceps, Mar.: 71–72.

Brooks, P. M., 1987. Back pain in the workplace. Med. J. Aust., 147: 257–258.

Charlton, K. H., 1988. Approaches to the demonstration of vertebral subluxation: 1. Introduction and manual diagnosis: A review. J. Aust. Chiropr. Assoc., 18: 9–13.

Chiba, S., Ishibashi, Y., and Kasai, T., 1994. Perforation of dorsal branches of the sacral nerve plexus through the piriformis muscle and its relation to changes of segmental arrangements of the vertebral column and others. *Kaibogaku Zasshi (Acta Anatomica Nippon).*

Damasio, A..R., 1994. *Descartes' Error: Emotion, Reason and the Human Brain.* Papermac edition, 1995. Macmillan, London.

Friberg, O, 1983. Clinical symptoms and biomechanics of lumbar spine and hip joint in leg-length inequality. *Spine,* 8: 643–51.

Ganora, A., 1984. Chronic back pain: diagnosis, treatment and rehabilitation. Patient Management, Aug.: 55–79.

Giles, L. G. F., and Taylor, J. R., 1985. Low-back pain associated with leg-length inequality. J. Aust. Chiropr. Assoc., 15: 135–145.

Grundy, P. F. and Roberts, C. J., 1984. Does unequal leg-length cause back pain? Lancet, iv: 256–8.

Heere, L., 1986. The spine in sports. N.Z. J. Sports Med., Dec.: 90–92.

Henderson, I., 1985. Low back pain and sciatica: evaluation and surgical management. Australian Family Physician, 14: 1149–1159.

Hoppenfeld, S., 1976. Physical examination of the spine and extremities. Prentice-Hall International, Inc., Englewood Cliffs, New Jersey.

Jensen, M. C., Brant-Zawadski, M. N., Obuchowski, N., Modic, M.T., Malkasian, D., and Ross, J. S., 1994. Magnetic resonance imaging of the lumbar spine in people without back pain. New England Journal of Medicine, July 14. 331, No. 2: 69–73.

Kapandji, I. A., 1974. The Physiology of the Joints. Volumes I–III. Churchill Livingstone, Edinburgh.

Kendall, H. O., Kendall, F. P., and Wadsworth, G. P., 1971. Muscles, Testing and Function. 2nd edition. Williams and Wilkins, Baltimore.

Knott, M. and Voss, D. E., 1968. Proprioceptive Neuromuscular Facilitation. Harper & Row, New York.

Kolata, G., 1994. Study raises serious doubts about commonly used methods of treating back pain. New York Times, July 14, 1994, p. A9 (California edition).

Laughlin, K., 1989. Low back pain: review and prescription. In Is our future limited by our past? Freeman, L. (ed.). Proceedings of the third conference of the Australasian Society for Human Biology. The Australasian Society for Human Biology, University of Western Australia.

Littler, T. R., 1983. Low back pain. Update, May: 59–73.

Loeser, J., 1996. Back pain in the workplace. *Pain,* 65:7–8.

Macquarie, 1981. The Macquarie Dictionary, 2nd edition, revised 1987.

Maitland, G. D., 1986. *Vertebral manipulation,* 5th edition. Butterworths, London.

Matheson, G. O., Clement, D. B., McKenzie, D. C., Taunton, J. E., Lloyd-Smith, D. R., and MacIntyre, J. G., 1987. Stress fractures in athletes: a study of 320 cases. *American Journal of Sports Medicine,* 15: 38–57.

Murtagh, J., 1983. Examination and diagnosis of low backache. Australian Family Physician, 12: 322–328.

Murtagh, J., Findlay, D., and Kenna, C., 1985. Low back pain. Australian Family Physician, 14: 1214–1224.

Porkert, M., 1974. The Theoretical Foundations of Chinese Medicine: systems of correspondence. MIT Press, Cambridge.

Rainville, J., Sobel, J. B., Banco, R. J., Levine, H. L., and Childs, L., 1996. Low back and cervical spine disorders. *Orthopedic Clinics of North America,* 27 (4): 729–746.

Rock, B. A., 1988. Short leg—a review and survey. J. Aust. Chiropr. Assoc., 18: 91–96.

Saal, J. A., 1988. Rehabilitation of football players with lumbar spine injury (part 1 of 2). The Physician and Sportsmedicine, 16: 61–68.

Schwarzer, A., 1996. How to investigate the patient with low back pain. *Modern Medicine of Australia,* August, 108–112.

Soukka, A., Alaranta, H., Tallroth, K., and Heliovaara, M., 1991. Leg-length inequality in people of working age. *Spine,* 16: 429–431.

Travell, J. G. and Simons, D. G., Volume 1, 1983; Volume 2, 1992. *Myofascial Pain and Dysfunction: The Trigger Point Manual.* Williams & Wilkins, Baltimore.

Twomey, L. T., 1974. Low back pain. Proceedings of a conference on low back pain held at the W.A.I.T. Bentley Campus, Sept. 14–15. School of Health Sciences, Western Australia Institute of Technology.

Twomey, L. T., and Taylor, J. R., 1994. *Physical Therapy of the Low Back.* Edinburgh, Churchill Livingstone.

Vernon, H., 1996. The role of joint dysfunction in spinal myofascial pain. *Journal of Musculoskeletal Pain,* 3: 99–104.

Wells, K. F. and Luttgens, K., 1976. Kinesiology: Scientific Basis of Human Motion, 6th edition. Saunders College, Philadelphia.

Further reading (annotated)

Achterberg, J., 1985. *Imagery in healing: shamanism and modern medicine.* New Science Library, Boston and London. A very readable introduction to *psychoneuroimmunology,* the study of the interactions between "mind" amd "body," and an analysis that will change your understanding of the patient-practitioner relationship forever.

Benson, H., 1976. *The Relaxation Response.* Collins, London. This very small book is a minor gem, condensing a great deal of technical research into meditation and similar practices.

Damasio, A. R., 1994. *Descartes' Error: Emotion, Reason and the Human Brain.* Papermac edition, 1995. Macmillan, London. I have mentioned this book above in the *References* as well. For me this was the most influential book I read in 1997—in its entirety it is a thoroughly persuasive argument for doing the kind of stretching exercises I advocate (especially the C–R aspect), although that is far from Damasio's original intention. I wish that Wilhelm Reich could have met Antonio Damasio.

Foss, L., and Rothenberg, K., 1987. *The Second Medical Revolution: From Biomedicine to Infomedicine.* Shambhala, New Science Library, Boston & London. The "infomedical" model locates the human being in an ecological, social and psychological framework with important implications for treatment of illness and analysis of "cause"—especially the degenerative diseases of our times—while preserving the deep insights into process provided by the scientific world view. The model can be fairly described as revolutionary in the Kuhnian sense.

Juhan, D., 1987. *Job's Body: A Handbook for Bodywork.* Station Hill Press, New York. This wonderful book examines (in addition to much else) the relation between anatomy and the *experience* of living.

Poliquin, C., 1997. *The Poliquin Principles.* The Dayton Writers' Group, Napa, California. Far and away the best book ever written on strength training. You will need to have someone at your gym explain what terms like "EZ French Press" mean, however.

Selye, Hans. *The Stress of Life*, revised edition. New York: McGraw-Hill Book Co. 1956, revised edition 1976, paperback edition 1978. The book that started a major new field of research, and it remains completely relevant today.

Quick Reference